30 DAYS TO
BETTER
HEALTH

THE EASY-PEASY WAY

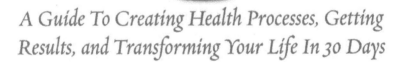

A Guide To Creating Health Processes, Getting
Results, and Transforming Your Life In 30 Days

PAUL KINDZIA

AUTHOR OF *SECRETS TO BREAKTHROUGH WEALTH*

30 Days To Better Health The Easy-Peasy Way

A Guide To Creating Health Processes, Getting Results, and Transforming Your Life In 30 Days

Copyright © 2018 by Paul Kindzia, Inc.

www.paulkindzia.com

ISBN-13: **978-0692997673**
ISBN-10: **0692997679**

Published by Paul Kindzia, Inc.

Printed in the United States of America

Cover Design – **Thomas McGee**

Editing – **Angela Kindzia**

For other queries, contact:

questions@paulkindzia.com

Disclosures

By reading this book you recognize that this is for education purposes and there are no guarantees for specific health and wellness results. By law, we cannot guarantee your specific results. You agree to not hold us liable for any results, good or bad, that you get from our informational and education content. You alone are responsible for your outcomes in life.

We do not believe in rapid weight loss, fad diet schemes, or overnight success programs. We believe in hard work, adding value, servicing others, processes, learning, adapting, and overcoming obstacles that stand in our way between where we are in life and what our goals are.

Please note that nothing within these pages, on any of our websites, videos, or any content or curriculum is a promise or guarantee of specific individual results. We cannot offer any specific meal plan, medical, allergy or disease advice on an individual case by case basis within this content. Any health numbers referenced are illustrative of concepts only and should not be considered average results, exact results, or promises for actual or future performance.

Paul Kindzia, Inc. is not a licensed medical practitioner and thus cannot give medical advice on an individual or case-by-case basis.

Making health decisions based on any information presented should be done only with the knowledge that you could experience significant health changes. Use caution and seek the advice of qualified professionals when attempting any lifestyle change, weight loss opportunity, or chronic disease remedy. Check with your own medical doctor, physician, or professional advisor before acting on any information.

This concludes with all the regular legal mumbo jumbo, disclosures, and disclaimers. We look forward to serving you with the highest standard of integrity and transparency. We value the trust that you put forth with us.

For additional valuable information including free resources, please visit our website at:

www.paulkindzia.com

Most people never achieve optimal health. Poor personal health and wellness contributes to low energy levels, low self-esteem, chronic diseases, daily stress, and unhappiness in life. It can also lead to financial problems as health care costs escalate. We teach proven health processes based on timeless principles that results in happier, more fulfilling, and balanced lives. We laugh a lot too.

ACKNOWLEDGEMENTS

Thank you to my family. It's one thing to repeatedly state, proclaim, yell, shout, preach, and grandstand that your most important investment is in yourself, your body, and your health. It's another to walk the walk and arrange one's affairs to live that philosophy yourself day after day. It would be impossible to eat, sleep, exercise, rest, recharge, push myself, learn, work, read, observe, travel, consult, write, produce, and get through the days without the unending support that it takes to fuel the machine. I am so fortunate and grateful for my wife Angela Kindzia and, "the pit crew" that keep me on the race track loop after loop running full throttle. And when I bump the track walls or crash into others you bring me into the shop, bang out the dents, and apply a little polish with spit shine along with abundant elbow grease. Thank you. I love you tons!

"The hardest part of writing a book, is reading a hundred. But it's also my favorite part." – **Paul Kindzia**

TABLE OF CONTENTS

How My Quest For Health Began

Have you ever wondered if your best health days are years or decades behind you? Are you constantly feeling tired, sick, depressed, and physically unable to meet the challenges of the day to reach your dreams?

Have you ever looked at younger folks or kids playing and said to yourself, "I used to be able to do that?"

Have you ever felt stuck at a certain weight or fitness level and wondered how to breakthrough to a more optimum level?

Have you ever wondered what common denominators of success exist in other healthy individuals?

Are you worried about your escalating healthcare costs?

Hi. My name is Paul, and I'm a health and wellness advocate. In fact, I'm a lot like you in that I wanted to transform my health and live a better life for myself.

Like all health and fitness practitioners, I had to start somewhere, and truth be told, I often wish that I didn't have to start so far back towards the end of the line compared to others. Perhaps you feel this way as well. There were many times I wish I could achieve faster results and I bet you wish you could too.

Where I Started

It probably would help if we started out answering an important question that you may have which normally is something along the lines of, "Hey, I'm trying to get smart about my health and wellness but have some doubts about you. How do I know you don't work for the government or really make burritos for a living?"

Answer: First, don't ever knock burritos or master burrito makers themselves. But I digress. You bring up an important question and I commend your skepticism. You are showing signs of having a high probability of success with your ability to think for yourself. You will probably be a fast learner in getting ahead in life. But if you want to know more about me, here's a bit more about my story.

I really am a finance geek with an undergraduate degree in accounting and an MBA in corporate finance. I'm a Certified Public Accountant, Certified Financial Planner, and the CEO of a wealth management firm.

If a finance nerd who sat at a desk all day staring at spreadsheets and computers all day can get healthy, there is more than hope for you.

I learned that the brain does work like a computer running on software (when it isn't being hijacked by your crazy emotions). That was a revolutionary discovery for me. I taught myself to write new software for my brain and then how to run it. It sounds crazy but then again, that's all habits and behaviors are. Habits and behaviors are just the repetitious pre-programmed responses that we have which are based upon the information and knowledge that was given to us during our life experiences. If you could change the input, you can change the output.

But what about the results? How did this transform me? Why is it important to you?

You may not believe it, but at various points of my life, I was a stressed out, anxious, fat piece of crap with a large CPA butt. I felt hopeless. I felt like life wasn't fun. I didn't have very good relationships with people. I had high cholesterol. I had high blood pressure. I had an ulcer. I used to get a lot of headaches. I felt lethargic. I hated my job. I felt like my future was bleak.

I had another problem coming out of college early in my career. It was a total personal conflict. Here I was, Mr. CPA with a fancy-schmancy MBA so interested in money, personal finance, and personal freedom. I craved financial security. But there was the debt I was dealing with. I had student loan debt, auto loan debt, credit card debt, then the mortgage debt. If you were someone I knew back then, I probably would have owed you $20 bucks too for covering me at lunch or dinner a few times.

UHHHHGGGG!!!! I was so frustrated and confused. I didn't have a framework for success. I had no template or guidebook. I was navigating life completely blind and ignorant.

I just wanted to be happy. So I told myself certain things that impacted my behaviors. I told myself that it was ok to drink soft drinks because, "I deserved them and needed the energy from the sugar and caffeine." I told myself that I deserved to be happy, so I indulged in things that provided immediate gratification at the expense of my own long-term self-interest.

My first job out of graduate school was working at Ernst & Young, an international accounting firm. Our largest client in the Atlanta office was a global leader in the soft drink industry and the firm had multiple fountain drink dispensers on all floors of the office. ALL YOU CAN DRINK! There is no telling how much sugar and caffeine I was consuming on a daily basis. (By the way, all you can drink doesn't mean drink all you can...)

I would get home from work and tell myself that I deserved to sit on the couch and "relax" while watching TV and eat some good snacks. I ate fast food (lots of it). On weekends I told myself that I deserved a treat for working so much and having such a hard life, so I would reward myself with something special like a rack of ribs, french fries, and more soft drinks. After all, I was entitled to be happy, wasn't I?

But it got to the point where my life was unbearable. Something had to give. I was so unhappy even though I was doing the things that were supposed to make me happy. I was eating what they showed me on commercials. I was buying stuff at the malls. I was driving a nice car, living in a nice house, and I had comfortable furniture. If I didn't have the cash to buy something I wanted, I'd just use my credit cards. I told myself that I deserved nice things since I had such a hard life. I never realized that I was the one making my life so much harder than it had to be. But of course, I was clueless and under the hypnotism of modern society (and what I refer to as the forces of evil) and American culture.

But then I realized that I was paying attention to all the wrong things delivered by modern society and started re-programming myself and amazing things happened. I learned that I didn't need permission from anybody to rebel against everything that I was being told by society (and the forces of evil). And it made all the difference in the world!

I re-programmed myself on my money, my health, my relationships, and my time management. I also started pursuing things that actually had an impact on my long-term happiness. It wasn't always easy but I'm glad that I did it. I had to learn a lot and maybe you will have to learn a lot too. But that's ok. I had a ton of questions, you probably do too.

Here's the deal. I had to learn how to get my sh!t together.

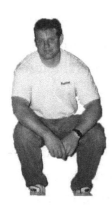

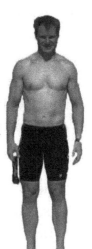

I had to learn how to go from a 220lb fat, unhealthy, anxious, unhappy CPA, to a 170lb bionic guy with boundless energy.

I had to get my sh!t together.

I learned how to change my health by re-programming myself. I went on to become a 13 time Ironman and multiple time marathoner.

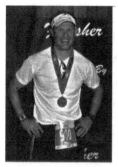

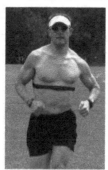

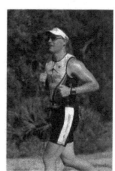

Now a lot of you might be saying, "Well I don't want to be an Ironman. I don't want to run marathons." I have GREAT news for you. You don't have to do these things at all to be happy, fit, and live a life of wellness (actually, it may be better that you don't do these extreme things if you want to maximize your health.)

You need to learn how to get your health sh!t together and you can do that by re-programming yourself the way I did. You do that by eliminating the bad information provided by the forces of evil and substituting it with the goodness that you can get here from me. And here's the good part – you can do this while having a job, family, friends, and living a fun life. There are plenty of people that have completely transformed their lives and you can too!

Now I know many of you will still want to say certain things to yourself and believe many things that were told to you by the forces of evil. Those forces are tricky and persuasive. They warped my stinking brain after all, so I know their power. I know this because I said many things repeatedly to myself based on that same crappy information that has been fed to you. I told myself that I just wanted to be happy. I told myself that I love eating certain things. I told myself that I loved relaxing when not at work because I was too tired and worn out to do anything else. I told myself that I loved watching TV and deserved that joy and pleasure.

You may be just like I was where you want to transform yourself and be healthy and happy. But then there is this little part of you that just isn't sure of some of the stuff I may tell you because you are not sure if it will make you happier (and of course it requires change and that's scary stuff). Who wants to put in the work and effort to change if it doesn't deliver the goods? That would be a complete waste of time. Fair enough. I have some questions for you.

Which guy below do you think is really happier? The guy on the left who told himself certain things about what he thought he loved and would make him happy or the guy on the right?

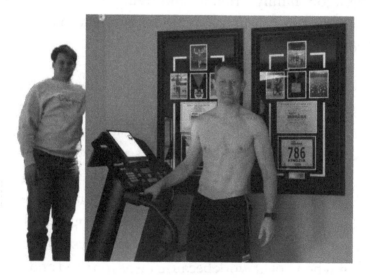

Which guy in the following pictures do you think makes more money and is more financially secure, the guy on the left or the guy on the right?

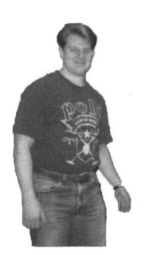 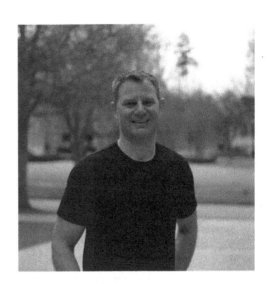

You must stop telling yourself the same lies that the forces of evil have been telling you.

Which guy in the next pictures do you think has more energy, has more fun, has better relationships, and has better control over his time? Which guy do you really think is happier across the board? Which guy has more confidence? Which guy is less stressed? Which guy is less anxious? Which guy feels better about the future? Which guy has better life experiences?

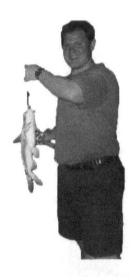 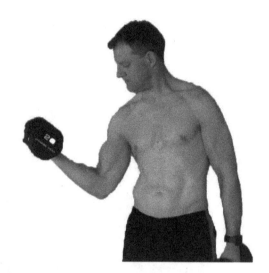

My before and after pictures aren't as important as what your before and after pictures are going to be. What do you want YOUR "after" picture to look like? What do you want YOUR life to look like? What kind of money do you want to make? How do you want to feel about yourself? This isn't as much about me as it is about YOU. What do you want from your life? How does it really feel to be the current version of yourself and how do you think it is going to feel when you roll out the new 2.0 version?

Look Out World, Here You Come

What you have a chance to discover is that your genetics don't have total control over you. Nor does it matter where you grew up, what city you live in, or where you went to school. You have an ability to learn and change.

Health Instructions Not Included At Birth

As many of you have realized by now, many of the important life skills aren't genetically pre-programmed in your brain at birth. Nor is our traditional educational system effective at providing you with essential life skills such as managing money, building quality relationships, or managing your own health.

On top of this, you are bombarded each day with food and lifestyle decisions that are not in your own self-interest but rather the interest of big corporations chasing profits.

"People are fed by the food industry, which pays no attention to health, and are treated by the health industry, which pays no attention to food." – Wendell Berry

Advertising is all around us and whether it is a pitch to save you time in your busy life or add pleasure, you are inundated with thousands of advertisements for pizzas, snacks, ice cream, alcoholic beverages, tobacco products, sugared cereals and other consumer goods that are bad for your health.

This takes you down the typical path that I experienced which is, "I work hard, am tired, want to be happy, and deserve this item which is an attempt at instant, but very brief, gratification."

The goal of this 30-Day process is to teach you how to alter your mindset and behaviors in a way that helps you become healthier and happier.

The interesting paradox of human behavior is that what we think makes us happy, often doesn't make us happy over the long-run. For instance, we may want a pizza and beer, or a piece of chocolate, or a bowl of ice-cream to make ourselves happy in the moment. But then ask yourself, if everybody is so happy in our culture behaving this way, why are millions of people unhealthy, experiencing chronic diseases and on prescription medications for anxiety and depression?

Does sitting on the couch, eating poorly, never exercising, drinking alcohol, smoking cigarettes, or taking drugs really make people happy? Because if it did, we'd have 320 million happy-campers in the United States.

But that isn't reality. Consider the following:

- Suicide is the 10th leading cause of death in the United States. Each year about 45,000 individuals die by suicide.
- For every suicide, 25 individuals attempt suicide.
- 35 percent of men and 40.4 percent of women are obese in the United States.
- Over 100 million Americans have diabetes or prediabetes per the CDC (that's about 1/3 of our population).

- About 75 million American Adults (1/3 of the population) have high blood pressure.
- 610,000 people die of heart disease in the United States every year (CDC)
- Approximately 40% of men and women will be diagnosed with cancer at some point during their lifetimes (National Cancer Institute)
- Chronic diseases are responsible for 7 of 10 deaths each year (CDC). Those are self-inflicted, non-natural-aging, early deaths.

Do you believe that all this sickness leads to happiness? Do you believe that the instant gratification items that you eat, drink, smoke, and ingest are the paths to happiness? Is it working for you? Is your life happy? Are you at peace with yourself? Do you feel rested, energetic, playful, engaged, and happy with your life?

The goal of this 30-Day journey is to help you discover how to build a better path to health and happiness for yourself in addition to helping others who want similar goals. One of the quickest and most efficient ways of accomplishing goals for yourself is to model your efforts after others who have already figured out how to make something work for themselves. Modeling success is tremendously valuable as you don't have to re-create the wheel and spend time and effort through trials and failures that will only increase the odds of you quitting before accomplishing your goals and objectives.

Your life is just one big ongoing experiment and laboratory as it allows you to see what works and what doesn't work. You must be honest with yourself and assess if your life is going as planned or if you feel content with your current situation. That's what successful people do, they assess, adapt, make changes, and try new alternatives until they reach their objectives.

Honesty and transparency is key to your success. Look around you. Look at the people that surround you at work, at home, in your social circles. Are most of those people healthy and happy? Health is one thing that is very hard to fake. Even tailored clothing can't hide muffin tops, beer bellies, double chins, labored walking, blood-shot eyes, ragged skin, and dark circles around the eyes.

Take note and start tracking common denominators of success and failures in your life. Search for consistencies and similarities amongst others that you want to emulate.

Becoming Your Guide

Over the years, I learned a lot of lessons on health and wellness. Now, after well over two decades worth of experience, I'm at a much different place than I was when I started out. Along the way, there were many health concepts I learned and acquired that can help any person desiring better health and wellness. I hope to guide you through some of those concepts as you progress on your own journey.

Maybe you are just starting out and don't know what to do. That's common. When most of us start out, we don't know many other wellness practitioners whom we can learn from. Fortunately, there are specific steps and action items that I can help you focus on.

Maybe you have mastered a few health concepts but want to progress to a higher level. There is always a higher level of health that is attainable.

I can relate to all those questions and uncertainties. There is a tremendous amount of knowledge to learn, and it's hard to sort through much of the noise. Plenty of people are trying to sell you short-cuts, fad-diets, and supplements. Health isn't something that can be immediately acquired by a pill, potion, or lotion.

If you feel stuck where you are, I can relate to that as well. There were plenty of times that I found myself stuck at a certain level of health and wellness and had to figure out how to get out of that phase and navigate around an obstacle. I'm still learning how to climb to higher levels and I'm still discovering new tricks, techniques, tools, and tactics to get me there.

The learning and journey will not stop; it will simply evolve because there are always new things to learn about your mind and body and how they both respond to stimulus.

As much as I am a "do-it-yourself-er," I still needed plenty of other people to help me along the way.

I needed books written by those eager to share their knowledge and experience. I needed the magazines and online articles. I needed and found value in blogs of people whose journey I found interesting and similar. I needed and found plenty of additional learning courses.

And now I feel obligated to distill what I've learned and pass on what I've learned (and where I've failed) to others who also want to achieve better health.

Writing is something that I love, but in an odd way it often feels strange for writers to share their thoughts and knowledge. Writers all have that fear. Who am I to share opinions and knowledge with others? Who will listen? What if people don't like what I have to say?

I've felt those fears myself. But I also realize how thankful I was for others who took the time to write out their thoughts and experiences, and in that same spirit, I believe that there are those who will find my words helpful to them.

If you have fears, doubts, confusion, or wonder if you could move up the health and wellness ladder, I can tell you with certainty that it is possible. It doesn't matter where you came from or where you started. The rules and principles of health and wellness are universal.

That's not to say that being healthy is always easy. It's not. But for those that put in the effort, the journey is better than the alternatives. My preferred saying is, "The juice is worth the squeeze." People that are healthier are happier. I never once met a person who proclaimed, "I wish I was sicker, so I could just stay home and lay in bed all day and not do anything in life that is fun."

When times get hard, when you get tired, when you have failures, when you feel alone and missing out on other experiences, have faith. Although there is a certain amount of randomness to many parts of life, you can control far more than you realize.

Periodically it is important to take the time to observe and acknowledge what happens if you don't take care of yourself health wise. Nobody else is going to do it for you. So many people find themselves without their health in the later stages of life. This leads to increased health costs, lost work, lost opportunities to do fun things with others. The only thing in their pockets is a list of regrets. One of those regrets is usually, "I wish that I had not been so stupid and wasteful with my one and only body."

There is a huge downside to health negligence. Do yourself a big favor: Acknowledge it. Accept it. Run away from negligence. If you ignore your health, it will ignore you.

In any case, I hope you find the following nuggets helpful on your path to health success and a happier and more fulfilling life. Please note, there is no way to teach over 25 years' worth of experience in a 240-page paperback book. That would be an impossible task.

This book is a compilation of short chapters designed to be implemented over a 30-Day time-period that address the key principles and obstacles that you are likely to encounter along your journey. Successful health practitioners execute these fundamentals, principles, and habits repeatedly. These are the foundations to success. Many may even appear to be common sense. However, common sense often does not mean common practice.

The chapters are assembled in a particular order that you may find helpful as you proceed through the book. Depending on where you are along your journey, your life experiences, and health history, not every topic or chapter may resonate with you at this moment. But it is likely that you will eventually progress through these issues and items on your own individual and personal timeline in life. When that time comes, I hope you will refer to this book repeatedly.

The information in this book is not formatted as a textbook based upon theoretical knowledge. Nor is the information an encyclopedia of complex and technical jargon that confuses people. The book is a compilation of very practical and useful approaches to the action items that matter when it comes to improving and maintaining your health and wellness. The objective is for others to make improvements in their life through better personal habits without having to go through all the heartaches and frustrations that I had to navigate. It's not necessary to become a medical doctor or obtain advanced degrees in physiology or nutrition to improve your life. The statistics back that up. You can do it and I hope this book helps you along your journey.

Have you ever wanted something so badly that you can feel your body and muscles getting tense just thinking about it? That's how it can feel with health and weight loss pursuits for many individuals. It is frustrating to want something so badly in life but not have the tools, resources, or knowledge to get there. Wellness is something that many people want desperately, yet it seems to elude the vast majority of the population.

Earlier in our lives and careers, that is often our situation. You want something tremendously, but you feel like you are stuck in the middle of a giant life riddle without the answers. Confusion results in a high amount of pain and frustration. It is the source of angst, turmoil, and teeth-grinding migraine headaches.

Where To Turn?
What most unhealthy individuals discover regarding wellness is that, "instructions are not included at birth." Or at least, you won't find them from the traditional sources of information,

like family, friends, and public education institutions. In fact, wellness is a puzzle and a riddle. The answers are always right there in front of you, but you can't pick them out. Wellness revolves around a lot of common sense, but unfortunately applying common sense is surprisingly uncommon in real-world situations. Humans are a flawed species with many behavioral issues and quirks.

What is often the most frustrating to unhealthy individuals is the speed of the process (or lack thereof), as it seems to take longer than most people prefer. If you're like most, you probably want to be healthy and fit RIGHT NOW. Information is great, but what about the results and transformation? That is what you are after. You want the fast solution that will change your life from frustration to contentment.

Feeling Your Pain

When you are unhealthy you often experience a significant amount of internal pain which is the result of wanting an increased level of health, and having a genuine desire to go after it, but then running into various obstacles that stem from the issue of "what to do now?"

Healthy and fit individuals aren't content just sitting on the couch and watching TV hoping that their lives will mysteriously and miraculously change. Healthy people are willing to make the efforts to change the course of their lives, and pursue the struggle from one obstacle to the next. Although they struggle, they consistently evolve.

As President Clinton once said, "I feel your pain." Although you don't know if he did or didn't feel your pain, if you are aspiring to achieve better health, seeking to move to higher levels of health, then there is no doubt about the pain that you feel.

This book is assembled with your pain and struggles in mind and the knowledge that will be required for you to progress. As you triumph over the pains and obstacles, you will generate incremental results. They will not always be smooth, but they should occur based on your skills at implementing the foundations and proven processes of health improvement. Over time, these incremental results will continuously transform you as an individual.

You will not always see or feel this transformation happening in your life. But others will. It's like being a parent. You won't see the daily changes as your child grows up but periodically others will proclaim, "Oh my, little Joey is growing up fast!"

Building Your Foundation

In this book, you will learn about the many obstacles that you will encounter as you change yourself from the inside-out. You will learn what core knowledge is needed to progress continuously throughout life so that you AUTOMATICALLY do the important behaviors and processes every day, every week, every month, and every year of your journey.

You will learn how to execute on the fundamentals of health and wellness and you will improve your efficiencies and have more energy. You will connect with fellow healthy and active individuals and people who can assist you. You will learn what to look out for and identify key success factors in different personalities. You will find yourself discovering opportunities to increase your energy and set up your life situation so that you don't get distracted by gaining more weight, developing chronic diseases, or by using ineffective methods that will cost you valuable time and energy.

As you improve your health based on solid fundamentals and proven principles of success, you will grow in all areas of your life. Steady progress will lead to more satisfaction and fulfillment even if the journey is challenging and hard.

Developing Habits That Lead To Success

If you learn the foundations of success described in the following chapters, you'll avoid a lot of mistakes, hold on to the fitness that you have, slow down the aging process and save precious time, all of which will allow you to improve your health at a faster and steadier rate.

Most individuals fail at being healthy because they lack the necessary core behaviors. They also lack correct processes. Most individuals or households will never achieve levels of health that are in line with their individual desires. Statistics back this fact up. Look at those around you in your communities and take note of how few people are living healthy and fit lives. There are reasons why chronic diseases are becoming a part of most households in the United States.

The best way to make sure you do the important processes every day is to make sure that your habits and behaviors are consistent with those that lead to healthy outcomes. Once your habits and behaviors are consistent with those that lead to success, you don't have to think about it so constantly or get distracted by too many decisions. Making choices and decisions will become much easier as they will be made automatically and by default.

It turns out that you perform the same routines each day because you are a creature of habit. You go through the same steps day after day. The trick to a healthy, fit, and energetic life is to figure out how to do the items that LEAD to wellness instead of doing those that keep you stuck in your ways or keep you sick and tired.

Steps To Success

Here is your action plan to get yourself to perform the important health and wellness processes every day so that you can make incremental improvements to your energy levels, body composition, confidence, and increase your upper limits of potential;

1. Become a lifelong learner. Education doesn't stop with high school or college; in fact, they are just the beginning. High school and college do not do adequate

jobs of giving you the information on what is truly important in life, namely health, wealth, and happiness.

2. Live each day based on principles of success. When you have proven principles to follow, you no longer find yourself aimlessly wasting your days wondering why progress isn't happening. We will discuss specific principles of health in upcoming chapters.

3. Don't get distracted and stay diligent. You can't do all the right processes and behaviors on Monday through Friday to then revert to poor habits on the weekends and expect long-term success. Health and wellness is a lifelong journey that requires a constant commitment to the core essence of the chosen path.

Start Now

The best time to start taking action in your life is RIGHT NOW. If you want the benefits of being at a higher level of health and wellness then you must start doing what it takes to get the information that you need, attract the people who can help, and obtain the health resources that it takes to get to that higher level.

You will find that writing important items down has multiple benefits. Begin by writing down important ideas and thoughts that you generate on increasing your health, habits that you need to create to improve your fitness, and principles that you want to follow with living at peace with yourself. Write these down in specific detail.

If you are going to start improving your health, write down how much weight you are going to lose, how much sleep you will get, and when you will do fun physical activities. Mentally visualize yourself being fit, healthy, attractive, and confident.

The more specific you can be, the higher the benefit during your execution. If you are trying to lose weight, be specific as to how much weight you will lose and by when, your stress levels, and your meal choices. Be specific.

Imagine the steps that are required to create new habits and behaviors. These habits and behaviors will pave the way to your path of health. You need to discover what processes must be developed and implemented, and then act on those processes.

Put actions and to-dos on your calendar, your phone, and your journals. Make processes automatic, such as walking and sleeping. Remind yourself each day what it is you are seeking to do – IMPROVE YOUR HEALTH.

Just because your life started with "instructions not included," doesn't mean that you can't obtain everything necessary to achieve your desired goals. You just need to assemble some individualized sets of instruction based on what you want to achieve. This book is designed to serve as the resource on the core instructions that you need for health success.

What's A Breakthrough?

break • through

noun

- A sudden, dramatic, and important discovery that leads to a large advancement or development in success resulting in a powerful transformation in personal health.

During your health and wellness journey, make it your goal to seek out and achieve as many breakthroughs as possible in as short of time frame as reasonable.

Health and wellness is not and will not be achieved in pure linear fashion. Life is never a straight path to any destination. Life is full of difficulties, triumphs, and failures along with plenty of periods of stagnation or personal plateaus.

Many people also have very distorted expectations on health, fitness, or weight loss goals. They often expect success to be an event that takes place where one is anointed and is accepted into the club with all the benefits of physical excellence. Rather than a step by step and cumulative progression, they want to believe that success kicks in overnight in one-fell swoop resulting in immediate transformation from sick and tired to superhero. That's not how the human body works so the quicker you come to terms with this, the better prepared you are to implement and execute on the principles that lead to long-lasting results. Wherever you are physically at the moment, it didn't take a week for your body to adjust and adapt to that state or level of health. Your body reflects the last 6 or 12 months (or years) of lifestyle behaviors. The good news is that excellent results can be achieved over just a few short months.

You may desire overnight success (who doesn't?) but the benefits of a long-lasting health protocol are worth it. You aren't going to get long-term health benefits by cycling through one fad-diet or exercise protocol after another if they aren't based on proven principles of success.

If we were to draw out and chart the health improvement expectations and dreams of many individuals, it would look like this:

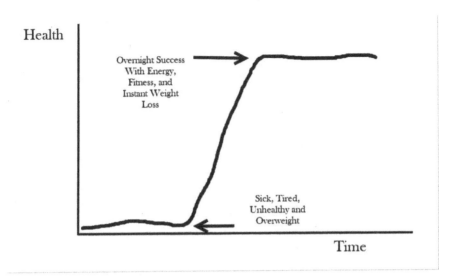

But we know that health and wellness isn't an overnight event. It's a lifestyle that keeps providing daily rewards. Success is earned over much longer periods of time, but the rewards last much longer as well. Thus, it could be quite useful to study those who have accomplished health success and seek out the common denominators of success.

One necessary and common denominator of success amongst healthy individuals who have changed their lives around is their ability to bust out of periods of stagnation and plateaus and experience what can be described as "breakthroughs." These breakthroughs are those moments in your life where knowledge, experience, and action all come together in a way that elevates you to a higher level of personal achievement.

Breakthroughs require effort. Breakthroughs require persistence. Breakthroughs require patience. But breakthroughs are the difference between success and failure and transforming your life. Without them, you will end up like most people who constantly spin their wheels but make no forward progress in life and are only left to wonder, "Why am I failing?"

If we were to draw out breakthroughs on a sheet of paper, they would look like this:

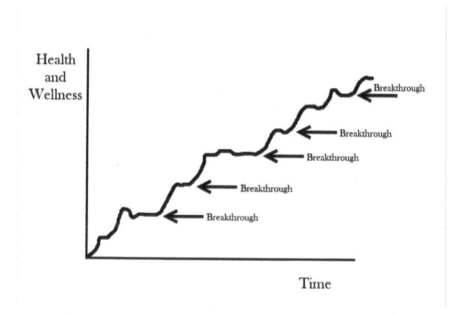

Breakthroughs are those moments where you bust through a period of stagnation or coming off a personal plateau where forward progress has slowed to a grinding halt. Plateaus are a natural part of life.

Part of mastery is practice and repetition and we could never master anything without practice and repetition. But how would you be able to master anything if you spent all your time trying new things and constantly implementing change? You would never be able to master anything if you failed to spend the necessary time practicing the fundamentals that were required with that stage of your personal development.

This is no different in any craft or activity. It applies to art, basketball, playing the piano, or learning math. Progress is never linear because you must spend ample time mastering certain skills before more advanced skills could be added to your repertoire. That's why bouncing from one fad diet to another without any lasting success is a failing method to health and wellness.

This book is about laying out the foundations of health building in a way that when comprehended and implemented will lead to breakthroughs. These breakthroughs are what will transform your life. It won't always be easy. Some breakthroughs will take more time than others. But if you apply yourself and submerse yourself in the lifestyle, you will get positive results.

Day 1 of Easy-Peasy – The Tools Of The Trade

It's Day 1 of the "Easy-Peasy" health and wellness cycle. Your health and body transformation is **ready for kick-off!**

Today is about taking a few moments to learn the tools of the trade. These are the items that will assist you in reaching your goals and maintaining long-term success. The tools may vary for each individual but there are some basic items that I would recommend for everyone. It will take a bit of time to acquire and get familiar with the basics. That's ok. It's more important to just take baby steps and make little bits of progress each day and each week. The results will come in time if you keep making small improvements day after day.

I have a list of essentials that I just can't do without. These items would include:

1. <u>A Fitness Tracker/Watch</u>. These trackers are a huge asset in tracking and logging your workouts, weight loss, and daily activity levels. Used correctly, you'll be able to see first-hand how active you really are (and trust me, most people have little to no-idea how little they move around each day. They just move from the bed, to a desk, to a couch and repeat daily.) I prefer and use Garmin watches and fitness tools and have been using them for well over a decade. I wear a Garmin Vivoactive

watch which doubles as my everyday watch. It's waterproof, can link with heart rate monitors, and has a lot of features that I really enjoy. You may be an Apple lover and may prefer an Apple Smartwatch. Fitbit and Samsung also have some very nice devices. All of them will track your daily steps and sleep patterns which are both critical for health and wellness. My Garmin products also link and connect online with family and friends through the Garmin website, so we can compare activity and hold each other accountable for getting in our daily steps. Nobody likes to get beat by their mother (but she does beat me often – Go Mom!)

2. A "Smart" Fitness Scale. Scales have come a long way since your Grandma's spring-loaded bathroom scale. Fitness scales provide high-tech smart data such as your body mass index (BMI), bone mass, body fat, and weight. A smart fitness scale sends a harmless electric current up through your feet and through your fat, muscle, bone, and water and measures your body's percentages of each. This is of great value when you are changing your body composition. Even if you are trying to "lose weight" you may end up putting on 5 lbs. of muscle and lose 3 lbs. of fat. If you didn't know any better, you would think you were going backwards and might make the tragic mistake of abandoning the very foods and diet that are leading you towards the promised land because you started to become a head-case. Do a search at Amazon.com for "Smart Fitness

Scale" and you'll see plenty of options at various price points. If you want to get extra fancy you could buy a scale that integrates with your other health tools. An example of this would be using the Garmin Index Smart Scale which automatically connects with your Garmin account, phone apps, fitness watch and provides in-depth metrics. Follow your own financial budget and think about those upcoming birthday and holiday wish lists.

3. <u>A Tape Measure.</u> As you make fitness and health improvements, you will be so happy that you were tracking your progress along the way. You will not only visually see the changes occurring with your body, but you will also have quantitative proof of your progress as you measure. Do a search at Amazon.com for "Tape Measure Health" and you will see various brands of inexpensive tape measures that are just perfect for measuring your future progress.

4. <u>Phone Apps/Website Accounts</u>. There are numerous apps for your smart phone. Many are developed direct from the fitness products that you own (like Garmin Connect which works with my Garmin fitness watch and other devices). MyFitnessPal (Owned by UnderArmour) is an excellent health app that allows you to track your most important health metrics and customize them. It also can act as a complete food journal. Whether you want to use just the basics or go all the way, MyFitnessPal is the app of choice on my

smartphone. Garmin Connect is the free app that makes uploading data from your fitness tracker as easy as 1-2-3 for Garmin owners. Apple, Samsung, and Fitbit all have their own apps. Learn to use these tools as they make life so much easier once you get the hang of them. They store and archive your fitness activities such as steps, sleep metrics, and a whole host of other cool features. They are easy to use, fun to monitor, and eliminate the need to write things down on pieces of paper that will at some point get lost or ruined over your lifetime.

You'll be using these basic and easy tools each day and they will become a habit no different than owning and using a toothbrush or comb.

Now, as you will learn continuously throughout this book, you won't be able to just snap your fingers and have all the above items ready to go in 15 minutes. **It's also important to note that it is NOT necessary to have any or all of these items to begin your journey and get started on your way to better health and fitness.**

It usually takes time for people to obtain and begin using these items. That is normal. These are the basic tools that I and many others use on our health journeys that have assisted us in achieving breakthrough improvements in our health and fitness. Once you get going, you will be unstoppable! Your mirror isn't even going to recognize you.

One final piece of advice on this topic of acquiring health tools. There is a BALANCE between what you want/need and what you can afford. I'm a finance guy at heart. I believe financial security is a HUGE component to health and wellness. I know through my financial practice that when people are stressed about money, have too much debt, and don't know how they are going to make next month's bills, they behave differently than those who are rock solid financially.

Our mind, body, and spirit are all connected. Our mental health impacts our physical and emotional health. When people are stressed about money, they are FAR more likely to binge eat, drink alcohol, consume processed foods, eat sugar or try to make themselves feel better by hiding from the world with pizza, ice-cream, beer, and potato-chips (or far worse).

Why do I bring this up currently? Because you are probably REALLY excited about making progress and jumping into your new health pursuits. You may be in what I call, "consumer heat" and ready to spend money on gadgets and tools that might not meet your budget constraints.

Know this; you can lose weight, be fit, and improve your health without ANY gadgets, fancy watches, electronic scales, and phone apps. These are just modern-day tools that didn't even exist a decade ago. Think about it, does that mean that no human beings were healthy in the last 10,000 years before technology took over? Of course not.

Be reasonable. Follow your budget. Don't ignore your finances. There are plenty of great investments that can be made in your health that do in fact cost money. The key is to allocate your financial resources in the most efficient and effective way.

Be financially fit, be physically fit, be mentally fit.

I post various articles on my blog about health, money, relationships, and happiness at www.paulkindzia.com I am here for you and want to see you achieve your goals in spectacular fashion. You can do it.

That's it for today. BOOM! Easy-peasy...

Day 2 of Easy-Peasy – Codename "M"

It's Day 2 of the "Easy-Peasy health and wellness 30-day cycle. Your health and body transformation is going to start getting in motion soon so buckle up.

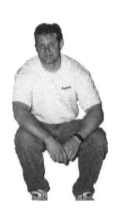

I had to learn how to go from a 220lb fat, unhealthy, anxious, unhappy CPA, to a 170lb bionic guy with boundless energy.

I had to get my sh!t together.

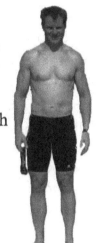

I can't tell you how many times I have been asked, "How did you go from the guy on the left to the guy on the right?" Sure, people were interested in my progress, but not nearly as interested as they were when they learned how they could do this for themselves. I just had to teach them about a secret ingredient to my success. Once you figure this one thing out, everything will fall into place and the results will just take over.

But before you dive in and go crazy with all your potential, there is a super-secret ingredient in the process of achievement and in the pursuit of personal excellence. The super-secret ingredient is codename "M." It's the key ingredient in recipe's workouts, processes, and routines. If you don't have the "M" in your arsenal of tools, everything is almost sure to fail over the long-term. Without it, nothing great can be accomplished, sustained, or maintained over the long-term.

What is "M" you ask? "M" is for "**MOMENTUM**." Everything you do needs "M" as the base ingredient in pursuit of health and wellness. Once you learn how to apply "M" to health and wellness, you will learn how to apply it to many other important areas of life. It is a game changer and that's why we will talk about "M" over and over again throughout the cycle.

You are in this transformation for the long haul. You aren't about to begin a fad diet or a temporary exercise routine. You are creating an all new "**YOU**" from the inside-out that will get a little bit better each day. You'll always be learning, always be evolving, and always be adding to what you've accomplished in the past. You will progress and transform one small step at a time.

You see, long-term success in anything requires **consistency**. Pro golfers didn't get great overnight. They began just as bad as everybody else. They didn't know how to swing a club at one time. But through consistency and momentum, they ended up mastering the game. The same applies to a pro basketball player, or piano player, or any high-level performer. The only way to get good at something is to practice it over a long period of time making small improvements along the way.

Now many people say, "Yeah, but I just want some fast results! How do I make quick gains?" But those are the same people that burn out, flame out, and quit only to regress back to where they started (or even much worse). You aren't interested in being a flame-out or a quitter. You are interested in winning this game and you will win big when you apply "M" to your formula.

You want the awesome and outstanding benefits of making changes that will last a lifetime. Once you start implementing the **core elements of success**, you will be amazed at how the results just naturally follow and become easy to maintain. People will start asking **YOU** for the secrets of success.

Momentum is all about starting with something small. Sometimes even super small. You may even start so small that people wonder, "What's the point?" But the point is that the key to long-term success is **consistency** and the only way to do something consistent over a lifetime is if it becomes a habit.

You will want to create habits that are so strong, natural, and easy that it will be no different than brushing your teeth or taking a shower. When habits take over, there is no more thought required to do something. It just happens automatically. There is no resistance when something becomes automatic.

Momentum then is like a snowball. It starts out small. But as it starts rolling downhill, it picks up speed and power. It just keeps growing until the energy is unstoppable. You never want to get in the way of something that has momentum, whether it is a monster snowball or a fast-moving freight train. But even the freight train had to start out barely moving and note how much energy it takes to get momentum going on a freight train. But then you can't stop it! That's what you are doing for yourself. You will be making yourself unstoppable through the power of "M."

Think about brushing your teeth as an example. When you were a kid, your Mom used to have to yell and force you to brush your teeth. That continued until it just became a habit. Then it became automatic. There was no more resistance. You don't even think about brushing your teeth anymore, it just happens subconsciously and automatically.

But wait, it gets better. When behaviors become powerful habits, you **FEEL BAD** when you **DON'T** do them! This is true even for people that have strong habits in eating healthy and exercising. If they DON'T eat healthy and exercise, trust me, they physically and mentally feel terrible. It bugs the crap out of them. They become cranky and suffer withdrawals.

Can you imagine that? Can you imagine becoming cranky and suffering withdrawals if you DIDN'T work out and eat healthy? But that is what is going to happen when you use "M" in your formula for success.

You are going to start with very small action items and at times they may even appear to be insignificant or too easy. But they are all designed to build momentum. Each day, you will improve upon something that seems so easy to do (because it was easy to do). But day after day, you just keep improving by 1%. Days become weeks, weeks become months, and months turn into years. 1% improvements just start stacking up like mountains and that is the magic of "M." You never take on anything that isn't sustainable over the long-term.

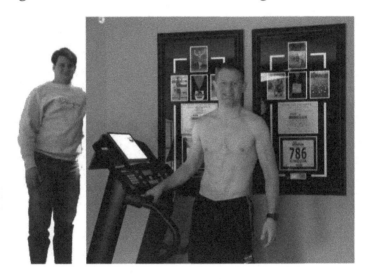

It's time you start visualizing your before and after pictures. What do **YOU** want to look like once you figure out how to implement "M" into your life? How is **YOUR** life going to change once you start developing habits that allow you to make very small 1% changes over time repeatedly? YOUR results will be just as amazing as mine or perhaps even better.

That's how you become a mountain of success. It's all from the magic of "M."

That's it for today. BOOM! Easy-peasy…

Day 3 of Easy-Peasy – The Principles Will Set You Free

Have you ever wondered how some people can achieve peak performance while others can't? Why some seem to have one breakthrough after another while others are constantly stuck in the mud and go nowhere?

To succeed, you need to learn how to get from where you are now to where you want to be in the future. It's about learning and implementing a process of achievement that is repeatable once you know what to do. That's what the 30-day health cycle is about. It's the "how-to" that allows you to get inspired to do more with your life and get the breakthroughs that you deserve.

Today is all about principles of success regarding health and wellness. Principles are fundamental truths that serve as the foundation for a system of belief or behavioral pattern.

Principles are timeless. And make no mistake about it, health principles are indeed timeless truths that have nothing to do with fad diets or some fancy exercise gadget that promises 6-pack abs if you make 3 easy payments by ordering a product right now.

Principles will allow your fears to diminish and be eliminated. One of the biggest fears in taking on any task or goal is the fear of failure. How do you deal with the uncertainty of something new? But here is the good news, principles give us guardrails to stay between on the road to success. If we follow the principles, then the road to success is straight ahead. You will just need to stay between the curbs.

What are the principles of health? There are 7 core principles that you will live by to gain momentum throughout your journey. They are:

1. Eat healthy
2. Exercise your body
3. Exercise your mind
4. Exposure to sunshine and fresh air
5. Get adequate sleep and rest
6. Reduce stress and anxiety
7. Avoid harmful substances (toxins, chemicals, drugs, alcohol, additives, and preservatives in foods.)

Having mastery over the 7 principles right now and all at once isn't critical because it is unrealistic. What is important right here and right now is just obtaining an understanding of what the 7 principles are so you could start building a framework of success necessary for growing "M."

Healthy individuals focus on specific objectives that encompass 1 of the 7 areas listed above. They move from one area to the next, balancing them out in a way that maximizes their health, wellness, and fitness.

Principles are the guiding force behind the objectives of your health processes which we will be covered tomorrow. Principles serve as the foundation for the systems you will learn to implement. They are the reasons to run your chosen "personal health software."

Principles guide your behaviors based on a mental chain of reasoning or thoughts whether you realize it or not. Thus, it is critical that you base your principles on your beliefs of what it is you want to be in life. You must know what it is you want to achieve and how you want to live your life.

Principles are based upon "what" you want to achieve, whereas the processes (discussed tomorrow) are the "how." There must also be a reason "why" you want to live life in a certain fashion. Super healthy people want to be healthy intentionally, not accidentally. That's what they want to do. It's important to them. The pursuit of health and wellness makes them happy (at least it should make them happy – if not, they are doing it for the wrong reasons.)

Principles act as your north star or your personal compass. They guide you in your personal pursuits. Principles should be at the core of your personal being. It's who you are. It's what your beliefs are. You should never compromise your principles based on the whims of the day or based on what others are doing or saying.

Of course, people all over the world live by different principles. Each of us may want different experiences in our lives and that makes the entire world a better place (for the most part).

Some people want to live an inactive life sitting around all day watching TV or playing video games. Some never want to learn or grow as humans. They make it mentally to about high school level and call it a day believing that they have enough knowledge to be happy and content. Many unhealthy and sick people just adapt to that status quo believing that there is no alternative and there is nothing to do about their health.

You will find people that want to sit around all day, eat pizza, drink beer, watch TV, and play video games. You will find people that want to smoke cigarettes or do drugs. You will find people that want to drink alcohol excessively. Some want to stay up all night and never see sunshine.

Healthy individuals want vibrant and energetic lives with physical activities. They want strong relationships, security with their finances, stimulating careers, and time for hobbies and passions.

When you decide what is truly important to you, you can live by principles of success that become the guiding light in your pursuit of excellence.

The Principles of Health and Wellness
There are 7 principles of health and wellness success. Health principles are timeless. They are like natural laws of the

universe. Health principles work in any time generation and they don't depend on fads or current thinking. These principles were true 1,000 years ago just like they will be true 1,000 years from now.

These health principles are non-discriminatory. They work no matter who you are or where you were born. They work regardless of your gender or your sexual preferences. They don't take notice of your religious beliefs or your political dogmas.

It doesn't matter if you are trying to improve your health or preserve your health. It doesn't matter if you have an exceptionally large income or a small income. These principles apply to all. Even if you are a high-earning celebrity or athlete, if you break these principles, your health will disappear on you in time.

Break these principles at your own risk.

If you need to, print off the 7 health principles. Put the list in your wallet, in a note file on your smartphone, on your mirror, and on your refrigerator. Everything we do will build off one of the 7 principles.

1. Eat healthy
2. Exercise your body
3. Exercise your mind
4. Exposure to sunshine and fresh air
5. Get adequate sleep and rest

6. Reduce stress and anxiety
7. Avoid harmful substances (toxins, chemicals, drugs, alcohol, additives, and preservatives in foods.)

"The journey of a thousand miles begins with one step."

– Lao Tzu

That's it for today. BOOM! Easy-peasy. The principles will set you free.

Day 4 of Easy-Peasy – Processes of Achievement

Yesterday we talked about the importance of living around the "<u>Principles</u>" of Success. Those principles are the "what" to do in life regarding your health and wellness. Today is about the "<u>Processes</u>" of success. Processes help us with the "how" to do what you need to do in life to be successful and reach your goals and objectives.

Think of it this way;

- Principles = What to do
- Processes = How to do it

Everything that you learn about health and wellness will be built around how to gain momentum with the principles of health. This builds off yesterday's chapter. It doesn't matter how small or insignificant your starting point is. What matters is if you make small tiny improvements day after day consistently and build "M." Remember, "M" is the secret. **Momentum is everything.**

You need to learn how to do more of what works and less of what doesn't. But people complicate things and set themselves up for failure when they take on more than they can chew. They try and change everything at once. It's too much of a shock to their system and they are trying so much at once that their body and mind can't keep up.

Whatever can't be done consistently eventually gets dropped. That's why people stop. They quit. They fail. Then they say, "See, I can't do it. I am just not cut out to be healthy."

But that is false. They just took on too much and too soon. They never implemented the timeless principles of health success. They didn't concentrate on "M" that would have changed their life for the better forever. Instead, they chased the fast track and continue chasing fad diet after fad diet and never experience true health or wellness.

The irony in all of this is that "M" doesn't make things harder and slower. "M" ends up making things easier and faster. Build "M" and there is no telling what you can achieve.

It makes no difference where you are starting out. It's all about building momentum from where you are starting and with time, you will reach your goals.

Software and Process Development

High level health and wellness practitioners execute personal practices that are far more effective than those of most individuals. One area of expertise that healthy individuals possess is in the area that can be described as "process." When you think of the term "process," I recommend that you imagine the word "software."

Software programmers write code based on a sequence of instructions that should be executed. For software to work properly, all steps necessary to complete the task must be included, and the instructions must be in the correct sequence for the software to provide the right outcome.

Health and wellness practitioners organize their life around personal sets of instructions that become so engrained in their daily behaviors that they perform those tasks automatically without much thought.

It is like brushing your teeth each night before heading to bed. You do this automatically without having to write yourself a "to-do" reminder note or follow a written set of instructions. You subconsciously and automatically brush your teeth in a certain way, moving your brush in a similar pattern, and similar time duration each night. You don't brush your teeth for 20 minutes one night and then 30 seconds the following evening. Nor do you subconsciously move your brush in a new direction or start in a different place each night.

You have built a process over time, and you execute the process repeatedly without conscious thought and effort. The behavior becomes automated. If for some reason you skipped brushing your teeth, something would make you feel awkward and even agitated. Skipping what is good for you (in this case brushing your teeth) would not make you happier, it would make you stressed or anxious because something would be ticking in your subconscious brain that something is amiss.

Imagine for a moment that you had a goal of getting in better physical condition to improve your state of health. To reach your objective, you will have to build processes and accomplish tasks specific to your desired outcome.

You might determine that the actions that could most greatly help you in becoming healthier would include exercise, nutrition, sleep, and stress reduction.

Becoming healthier now must include the building of processes (writing the software) that helps you complete daily tasks that are in line with your desired results that become automated and require very little thought and effort. Those processes just become part of you no different than brushing your teeth.

Developing Processes To Help You Commit

Let's start with exercise. You would begin by brainstorming different ways that you could complete more physical activities during the week. Examples might include:

- Lifting weights at a gym
- Swimming on your lunch break
- Going for a walk with your spouse

Let's take the first example – lifting weights at a gym. What are the actual physical steps required to make this happen in your day? They would include the specific tasks of:

1. Putting workout clothes in a gym bag
2. Putting the gym bag in your car
3. Driving your car to the gym
4. Walking from the car to the gym, into the locker room, and changing clothes
5. Getting on the workout floor
6. Executing a workout routine
7. Heading back to the locker room to shower and change
8. Exiting the gym

You may be reading this and be saying, "Duh, this is so basic and simple. How is this going to improve my health and give me the results that I desire?"

The difference between those that achieve long-term health success and those that are left only with hopes and dreams is that achievers execute the software every day. They complete every step, in the proper sequence. They follow their individualized written instructions of tasks that need to be completed to achieve results. They continue these daily tasks until they become engrained and automated.

They don't ask themselves how they feel and use feelings to dictate their actions. They don't wonder what else they could do that is more fun or relaxing. They don't imagine being at home watching television while eating a bag of chips. They don't get distracted daily by doing non-essential tasks that waste precious time. Rather, they run the software each day on the items that relate to improving their health.

Have you ever met a marathon runner or an Ironman Triathlete? They can do some amazing physical activities. Do you think each day the marathoner wakes up early and says, "I totally feel like getting out of this warm bed and going out in the cold weather and completing my training (running the software)?" That is not reality.

Marathoners, athletes, and professionals are all human. They like relaxing and resting as well as the next person. The difference is that they don't behave based on how they **feel** at any moment of the day. Rather, they behave and run the software required at that time of day to accomplish their desired tasks. They do these tasks until they become automated where they don't even think about "not doing their training."

At mile 18 of the marathon when their legs start to seize up, ache and hurt, the marathoner doesn't stop running and say, "My legs hurt. I want to go home and rest and eat pizza." Well, maybe they do, but I'm sure they quickly trump those distracting thoughts and then say to themselves, "You have a task and objective to complete. Run the software in its entirety (which includes crossing the finish line and obtaining the finishers medal)."

They complete all tasks in the proper sequence and then move on to the next required task (which may include eating a healthy pizza AFTER they accomplish their required tasks and objectives.)

Your objective today is to give thought into the processes that you must build and execute that is like personal software. In this way, each day of running that automated software will move you toward your desired objectives.

That's it for today. BOOM! Easy-peasy. These principles will set you free.

Daily Check-In

HOW DID YOU DO TODAY WITH YOUR GOALS?

- Are you starting to implement momentum into your daily health habits?
- Are you starting with small changes and building upon them consistently?
- Are you beginning to implement the principles of health into your life every day?
- Are you starting to build processes to implement the principles of health into your daily routines?

Day 5 of Easy-Peasy – Tracking Results

Day 5 is all about tracking results. One of the main goals of this entire journey is the transformation from your old self to your new self. You are going to be going from **OLD YOU** to **NEW YOU** and changing yourself from the inside out making lasting and permanent changes.

We aren't talking about just a little bit of change that nobody else will notice. That's rubbish. We are talking total super-duper mind-blowing changes to your health and wellness that will scream, "I've arrived in style!" This will be the kind of change that will make other people go, "Wow! I didn't think you had it in you." But more important than impressing others, you will impress yourself and feel like a million dollars because it feels **SOOOO much better** when you truly are healthy and energetic.

To achieve your goals and experience breakthroughs, you must make progress and improvements. How will you know if you are making the gains necessary to reach your goals if you don't track your progress? What should you track? The easy answer is, "anything that you feel is worth tracking that will assist you in assessing your progress and results."

We know the secret to success is "M." M is the **momentum** that leads to **consistency**. With consistency, you can do anything. The key to "M" is small attainable changes that just keep stacking up over longer periods of time. These aren't "turn your life upside-down changes that are too big and unsustainable." If something is unsustainable, then it can't and won't be consistent. And you won't be able to build "M" if you can't do something consistent. Remember, "M" is the secret sauce.

When it comes to tracking, you'll want to periodically take an inventory of your progress. This will give you the feedback that you are moving in the right direction little by little. Brick by brick, stone by stone, great pyramids are built. You are going to be like a great pyramid, built one brick at a time. Results won't be linear. You will have plateaus and even some setbacks along the way. That's normal. But nothing should stop your long-term "M."

You are welcome to track anything and everything that you feel is going to help you stay motivated and give you an honest assessment in your progress. Some of my favorite items to track would include (but are not limited to);

Tape measurements;

- Neck
- Chest
- Waist
- Hips
- Biceps (flexed of course – give us a gun show!)
- Thighs

- Calves

What I find is that consistency helps with tape measurements. Where you place the tape on your body part can make a difference in the measurement. I aim for the largest measurement in that area or I make special note of where I am placing the tape so that the next time I obtain a measurement, I am comparing "apples to apples."

Scale measurements;

- Weight
- Body fat %

Other measurements;

- Sleep metrics
- Steps taken per day (I aim for 10,000 per day minimum)
- Resting heart rate
- Blood pressure (No need to take daily but perhaps monthly. You can also buy your own blood pressure monitor at a drug store rather than going to your doctor's office.)

When you take measurements, it's important to take them at the same time and under the same set of circumstances. For instance, I like to take my measurements and weight first thing in the morning. I wake up, use the bathroom, and on an empty stomach obtain my metrics for the day. I find that my level of hydration or if I eat certain foods can impact my body fat % and even my weight itself because my body is holding water related to salt content levels in the food I most recently consumed. Some variations are normal and expected.

This may sound hard to keep track of these metrics. But with the tools I recommend, it really is easy and fast. I use the UnderArmour "MyFitnessPal" app and the Garmin Connect app to keep track of 80+% of my data (probably more). Most of it is either uploaded manually or automatically as part of my daily routine each morning (just like software – I run my processes). It's easy-peasy.

I also suggest you take some "before" pictures. Nothing will make you prouder than going back over time and looking at where you started versus where you are currently.

Keep in mind that you may like tracking some items daily like weight and body fat %. Other items like tape measurements may be better to do every 30 days or so. You'll find what works best for you. It's most important to just start somewhere and build the habit and the consistency that leads to "M."

If you email us at the contact page on www.paulkindzia.com and request a sample "Tracking Spreadsheet," we will email you one to get you started tracking your progress.

It's time to start getting some initial metrics down on paper for tracking.

That's it for today. **BOOM! Easy-peasy...** Tracking will help you stay on track to reach your goals.

Day 6 of Easy-Peasy – Eating Healthy

I have a story that I wanted to share that may seem hard to believe. At various points in my life, I was quite unhealthy. I was this guy:

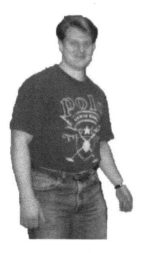

When I was in unhealthy physically, I can now look back and realize that I was also in unhealthy mentally and emotionally as well. Only through hindsight do I now realize how everything is connected in some weird and bizarre way with our body, mind, and spirit.

When I was at my unhealthiest, I had several beliefs that were firmly rooted in my mind. I was quite stubborn with these beliefs. I was also firmly against changing them for many reasons. In many ways, I kept holding myself back from getting the breakthroughs and transformations that I really wanted to achieve for myself.

During those dark times, any number of sources could have given me accurate information on what to eat or what to believe. They could have told me specifically to eat my vegetables no different than my mother did while I was a child growing up. But either I wouldn't listen or I wasn't capable of implementing that knowledge and information into my actual day to day life in a way that was consistent or sustainable. Long story short, I had nothing in place to build "M" in my life.

What I also had, but would never admit to anybody (even myself), was that I had some fear. I was afraid of the unknowns. I wasn't willing to do certain things because if I failed, what would that mean for me? I also didn't know how to help myself, so I did nothing instead. I just kept doing more of what wasn't working. Unhappiness bred more unhappiness. It was vicious circle.

I wanted to be happy no different than anybody else. I used food to make myself happy in the short run. The happiness was more like immediate gratification. When I was depressed, angry, stressed, anxious, or bored, I would eat foods that made me happy (at that moment in time). But oddly, the more of these foods I ate, the less happy I ended up with myself. I felt worse day after day. I had less energy. I was moodier. In a quest to make myself happy I was making myself unhappy.

I also had beliefs on certain foods. I liked certain foods and convinced myself that they were fine to eat. There was no shortage of advertising and promotion of these foods that I liked to eat; pizza, pasta, frozen foods, soda's, chips, and processed foods. They were easily obtainable, reasonable in price, and they tasted so good. They also provided short-term immediate gratification when I ate them.

I didn't like vegetables. I wouldn't eat vegetables. I didn't mind fruits but never really went out of my way to buy, keep them on hand, or consume them. I told myself that a life of clean eating sounded like no fun at all, boring, and unsustainable. Again, I had very deep-rooted beliefs.

I believed that certain foods were going to make me happy, so I ate those foods. They in turn really made me unhealthy and unhappy. Likewise, there were other foods that I thought were going to make me very unhappy, but only through time and success I realized that they make me very happy. It's quite bizarre if I think about it. I just wouldn't have believed it if I didn't experience it myself.

What if I told you that the foods that I previously loved and were addicted to are now foods that I wouldn't eat if you tried to force me to eat them? There is no way I would eat the stuff I ate back then. Not only do I know it's not good for me, but I wouldn't like the taste or how it would make me feel.

And what if I told you that if you tried to take my healthy foods away from me I would fight you tooth and nail to not let that happen. Those foods are my rocket fuel that I crave and depend on to keep me feeling energized, happy, and nourished.

What happened during this transformation? How did I switch from a garbage loving eater to a clean and healthy eater? I crowded out and replaced things slow and steady over time as I built "M." I didn't change everything at once. I didn't turn my life upside down.

I believe that is the main reason people fail on their quest to change their health permanently. They are given or have access to accurate knowledge and information. They are told what to eat. But here's the deal. If I told you to eat your fruits and vegetables and sent you on your way, how likely are you to use that to change your life? It's not likely you will succeed even if the knowledge and information is 100% accurate.

But it's not just the knowledge and information. It's the "how-to" portion in the process of achievement that makes the difference.

There is still plenty for you to learn about what to eat and what not to eat. You'll be amazed at how much there is to learn and how far down the rabbit hole you can go on almost any area of human nutrition. But none of that is important right now.

What is important is that you understand the basics of where you are and where you are headed. Then you slowly just crowd out and replace little by little, one thing at a time allowing your body to adjust along the way. You only take on what is sustainable so that you can consistently apply each step along the journey.

When you make small changes that are **sustainable**, then you can apply those changes **consistently**. If you can do anything **consistently**, you can build "**M**," (build MOMENTUM). With **momentum**, anything is possible.

"Never compare your chapter 2 with somebody else's chapter 14." – Paul Kindzia

If you can imagine how grade school works, they don't give a 3rd grader physics and differential calculus as the curriculum. If they did, the grade schooler would be sure to fail. It's no different in your path and journey to lasting health and wellness.

You must take things step by step, mastering one item before going on to the next. This should also give you confidence because you won't be flipping your entire life and habits upside down and all at once which would only lead to an unsustainable situation.

I want to share with you the most terrible, horrible, brainwashing belief statements that will 100% derail all your desired health breakthroughs. These statements are made by most and believed by many for several reasons. The two statements are often expressed in the form of a question and right now you may even believe these two statements:

1. Don't you want to enjoy your life?

2. What do you do for fun?

These two dumb-dumb duo beliefs can apply to most things that are bad for us; drugs like heroin or crystal meth, alcohol, marijuana, sugar, or unhealthy foods and snacks. Many people BELIEVE that they are living a more enjoyable life and having more fun by consuming things that harm them over the long-term. They believe that the pursuit and achievement of short-term gratification will equate to long-term happiness and fulfillment.

Doing harmful things to ourselves in the pursuit of short-term gratification doesn't lead to long-term happiness and fulfillment. Most people just don't have the initial courage to overcome their fears. They may not know how to change or what will happen if they do change. Will their friends still like them (maybe not!) Will people make fun of them (some will!)

You see, when you change into someone new, there is uncertainty involved. You don't and won't know exactly who you will become or what you will stand for (and against.) I did the exact same thing. That's why I resisted change for so long at the expense of my own self-interest.

But now I can tell people with full confidence and assurance through my own journey and experiences. Let me ask you a few questions as proof and review what was covered a few chapters ago for positive reinforcement. Who do you think enjoys their life more, the guy on the left, or the guy on the right?

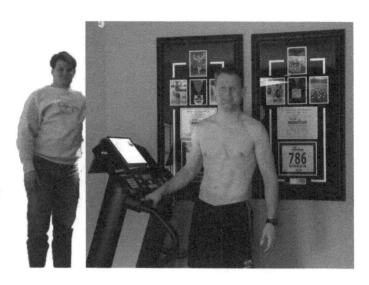

Who do you think has more fun in life, the guy on the left or the guy on the right?

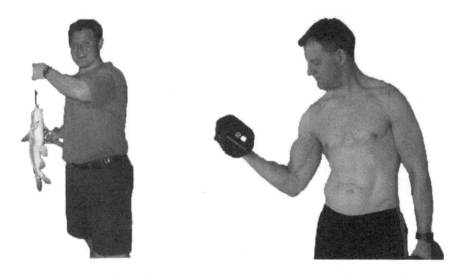

Who do you think makes more money and is happier, the guy on the left or the guy on the right?

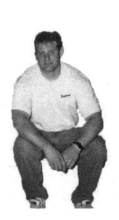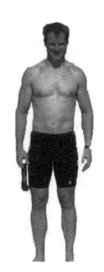

You must make some choices about your belief system just like I had to. What you believe will dictate your future course of action and your decisions. This comes down to choices and beliefs. What will you believe about the role of food in your life?

I wouldn't have believed it myself had I not experienced it first-hand. The foods I thought made me happy didn't end up making me happy. They made me unhealthy and unhappy. Nor did I end up having a lot of fun in my life when I ate poorly and was unhealthy.

The foods that I thought would make me unhappy, ended up doing the opposite. I enjoy healthy foods now. I crave them. I sometimes catch myself worrying about what would happen if I lost access to my healthy nutrition. Can you believe that? I worry about people taking my organic fruits and vegetables away from me. It's crazy!

There is an eating progression that you will have to embark on. You must learn to slowly substitute foods and eat more of what is good for you and less of what is bad for you.

THE GOOD	THE BAD
Vegetables	Processed foods and meats
Fruits	Preservatives
Nuts & Seeds	Chemicals like MSG or Aspartame
Legumes (Beans & Lentils)	Alcohol
Fish (Wild Caught)	Gluten
Healthy Grains Like Quinoa and Oatmeal	Saturated Fats
Healthy and Lean Meats (Grass Fed, Hormone & Antibiotic Free)	Trans Fats
Eggs (Pasture Raised, Hormone & Antibiotic Free)	Refined Carbohydrates (White Flour Type Foods)
Superfoods Like Cacao Mushrooms, Spirulina, Moringa, Maca, Wheatgrass, Turmeric	Sugar! Sugar! Sugar!

If you read a label and it has super long words that only a chemist could understand, it's not good for you.

When you open your mind, and embrace a different belief system, everything then becomes easy-peasy because you are no longer fighting the resistance.   You are sailing with the winds at your back.

The hardest part of this obstacle is just having the courage to do some honest self-reflection within yourself. You have to ask yourself, "I have been eating certain foods and behaving in certain ways. Did these methods produce success? Am I living the life I envision? Am I reaching my goals and objectives? Is eating like this really leading me to inner happiness?"

Many people are stressed, anxious and unhappy with themselves in life. They never search within to understand what is the true source of this discontent and unsatisfied feeling. Are you living a good life? Only you know the answer to that.

"If you don't know where you are headed, any road will take you there." – Lewis Carroll

That's it for today. You are making progress and moving away from the guy on the left and towards the new you on the right. You can do it. I know you can.

BOOM! Easy-peasy... Eating healthy will allow you to reach your goals and become healthy and happy.

Day 7 of Easy-Peasy – Daily Exercise

Today is one of my favorite topics and that is daily exercise. For most people, this is their least favorite and the one that makes them cringe the most. Who wants to suffer everyday while exercising and punishing their bodies? I think people are surprised when I answer that question myself with, "You don't have to suffer to be healthy."

Your goal will certainly be to exercise daily. But before we get into the details on that, let me share some great news with you. I know the reason most people fail at sticking to an exercise program. I know why people can have all the best intentions in the world. I know why people can come up with the greatest New Year's Resolutions imagineable on how they are going to start and stick with an exercise program. And then they flame out big-time. They flop. They stop. They quit. They fail. And then they break down and feel unworthy and helpless.

Little did they know that they were doomed to fail from the start. Little did they know that even with the best of intentions, they weren't going to last. They were missing the most critical component of success in their daily exercise program. The fact that they most often start out going full-on gangbusters just expedites their own demise. Then they feel like such a loser about themselves and it is unnecessary. If they only knew the missing critical component that would have made the process of achievement so much easier to implement.

Are you ready for what the missing component was? It was "M." The fact that they started out like gangbusters and tried to do too much and too soon just exponentially increased the probabilities of failure. They went down in flames like most people.

There are two components to an outstanding exercise program. They are:

1. Consistency
2. Workload

The most important component is the first one and that is consistency. Consistency must come first. It's far more important than workload, especially in the early stages of any new change in your daily routines.

I know you are familiar with Michael Phelps, the most decorated Olympian athlete of all time. Enough gold has been wrapped around him that he might start being confused with an Egyptian mummy like King Tut. Do you want to know what Michael Phelps did better than anybody else? He trained far more consistent than the others.

This allowed him to build "M" (momentum) and increase his workload a little at a time. He would train on Saturdays. He would train on Sundays. He would train on holidays. He would train on Christmas. He was consistent like no other.

But he and his coach knew something that the others didn't. They knew that little by little, month after month, year after year, they could slowly increase the workload.

When Phelps was 13, he was already swimming a lot. But not as much as he was swimming at the age of 15. By 17 years of age, he was outdoing his former 15-year old self. And by 21, forget about it. He could handle (and desire) higher and higher amounts of workload. He was smart and consistent about it. He used **momentum**.

But if you go back and think about it, he didn't try to do the swim practices that he was doing at 25 years of age when he was only 11. That would have been insane. His body wouldn't have been able to handle it. Sure, maybe he could pull it off for one workout. But he wouldn't be able to do it the next day and the next day after that. The workload would have been unsustainable which meant that he would have been inconsistent.

He would have needed large breaks to recover. Or he would have become injured because he was placing too much strain on his body. He also would have hated the process because he was over-extending himself. It would have led him to quit, give up, flop, fail, and maybe take up arts and crafts.

Remember this when you start a daily exercise routine. Yes, you need to start exercising every single day (for the rest of your life). But don't get too far ahead of yourself right now. It's far easier to implement than most people realize. I'm living proof.

You must assess yourself honestly and exercise based on a level that will allow you to exercise the very next day. Don't do anything that will wear you out or over-exert yourself where you can't back it up and repeat it the next day and the day after that. That means going far easier than most people start out. How can you not like easy?

Can you do one push-up from your knees? Can you do a single sit-up? Can you do a walking lunge or a squat with your own body weight? Can you walk a certain number of steps above what you would do in the normal scope of your daily routine? Great, that all counts as exercise.

Right now, don't even think about what exercise is going to look like a month from now, or a year from now, or ten years from now. That isn't important. You'll never get to a month from now, or a year from now, or ten years from now if you don't execute on the core principle of "M." "M" is all that matters right now. That's all you should pay attention to.

Can you wake up tomorrow and do a push-up, a sit-up, a squat, or walk some steps? Maybe go past the mailbox when you go and get the mail and then turn around and come back. Or, park your car a bit further away from your work building or grocery store to get in more steps.

How many times have you seen cars circling the parking lot over and over again, so the driver could get a closer parking space because heaven forbid them walk a few more steps? Did you park a little bit further away? Good, go to bed tomorrow night telling yourself the absolute truth – YOU EXERCISED! Mission accomplished.

The day after that, your head is going to hit the pillow and you are going to feel proud of yourself and know – YOU EXERCIESED! You are a winner. You are making progress on your goals and improving each day. You started building consistency. You are transforming yourself from the inside out. You are on the path to long-term sustainable success.

You are going to do this every day for the rest of your life. Don't make this hard or complicated. Don't over-exert yourself. Don't do anything physical that would make you miss the next day of exercise. It does not matter how small or simple you start.

Remember what we discussed above, there are two components to an outstanding exercise program; consistency and workload. And now think about all those people that start out gangbusters with all those wonderful intentions and resolutions. What happens to most of them within the first ten to fourteen days? They quit.

They fail at implementing consistency first. They try to implement a program that is not sustainable. Since it was unsustainable from the start, they never could harness the power of "M." They never gave themselves the chance to build momentum and succeed at their health goals.

But that is not going to be you. You aren't going to flame out and flop like those others. You are going to do this. You are going to win at this game. You know the secret. You know you don't have to go crazy in the beginning or anytime for that matter because you will limit yourself to what you could back up the next day. Isn't that comforting and encouraging?

You know that the most important thing to do right now as you get going is to work on consistency rather than workload. Every single day you are going to go to bed and say to yourself, "I DID IT! I EXERCISED!" You will wake up the next day with so much confidence because you know that you have a streak going. You will not want to break that streak. You are consistent. You are implementing a program that is sustainable. You are harnessing the power of "M."

Amazing things are going to happen. You will wake up one day and say, "You know what, I can easily do two push-ups today, and two sit-ups and two squats. I also can walk even further past my mailbox down the road." But you aren't going crazy and doing anything that wouldn't allow you to easily do the exact same workload the next day.

You certainly shouldn't go and try to max-out and see how many push-ups you could do to expedite immediate results. We know that doesn't work. When you max yourself out, your body breaks down. It needs recovery. It isn't ready to go the next day. You need time off. You burn out. You quit. Then you are like the others and start being inconsistent. You did things that were unsustainable.

The beautiful and wonderful thing about doing a program like this is that it is SO EASY-PEASY! It's so basic. You have the rest of your life to just inch things up consistently. And wait until you see the results over time. You are going to be blown away with the long-term results. How good is it going to feel when you look in the mirror and see that transformation with your own two eyes? How proud are you going to be a year from now, five years from now, ten years from now as the "M" just continues to build and you are consistent with the principles of success?

Here's the funny part. Many people will say, "That sounds like it is going to take forever to get the results I want." They won't do it. They will do it like everybody else and go gangbusters and pile on the super-sized workouts right off the bat. Then they will discover that their approach is unsustainable with no consistency and they flame out and fail. They will never accomplish their goals with the traditional approach to starting an exercise program. That's why people keep failing at this game and it's unnecessary.

Right now, it doesn't matter what you want to do for your exercise. I encourage you to keep it super simple and nothing complicated. A push-up, a sit-up, a squat, a lunge, some extra intentional walking steps. Maybe it is a bike ride, or a game of tennis.

I want you to implement "M" into your daily life. I want you to concentrate on the next 30 days. Don't worry about what exercise you'll be doing in a year or a decade from now. "M" will take care of the future. Just worry about consistency right now and making yourself proud for exercising every single day.

That's it for today. It's going to be EASY-PEASY if you harness the power of "M." Success is now in your future. You can see yourself winning at this. You can feel the **momentum**. Visualize how good it is going to feel with your body and your health in the future. WINNING!!!

BOOM! EASY-PEASY... Exercising daily will allow you to reach your goals.

Day 8 – Knowledge + Implementation = Progress

I've been fortunate to meet, build relationships, and learn from some very healthy and passionate individuals over the years.

Just like you, none of these people were born with all the knowledge that was needed to transform themselves physically and mentally. One friend of mine went from being an out of shape corporate finance professional with a penchant for alcohol to a world class Ironman triathlete. The transformation was nothing short of stunning.

Like many people, he hit rock bottom when he discovered that a high paying job alone was nowhere near the answer to a healthy and happy life. He knew at the bottom of his heart that he needed big changes. He was willing to turn the ship and begin on a new course in life, even if he didn't have all the answers.

Within a few years of starting his health and athletic journey, his happiness levels changed dramatically. There was a whole new person within himself. Everything changed when he made that commitment towards a lifestyle of health and wellness.

He made new friends, developed new habits, and went on a journey of educating himself on the truth about health and wellness. It was like a watching a personal supernova where his entire life was expanding. His life wasn't contracting, it was growing for the better in all areas of life and I was able to see this remarkable personal transformation with my own two eyes. It was inspiring and provided a personal example to myself that it is possible to make the needed changes within myself.

My friend had a college degree and a master's degree. He was an intelligent individual and a hard worker. But it wasn't one of those stories that you hear about where a person is this natural athlete that is good at all sports and goes on to easy glory. It was a story of a person who deeply valued self-reflection, truth, and learning. He loved knowledge, and he loved reading books and articles.

I also love knowledge and learning, so I admired that aspect of him, but I also wanted more of the results that he was obtaining in life. I swallowed my pride and asked him something that was bound to reveal a few of my personal shortcomings. I asked, "What happened that made the difference?" He said, "It's not just about the knowledge alone. The knowledge is required but only one component of the equation. You need the knowledge first and then it's about the doing."

"Success is steady progress towards one's personal goals." –
Jim Rohn

People are always asking me about how I transformed myself over the years because they want to experience that same transformation for themselves. They often ask me questions about what my keys to success were.

They are stunned when I show them either in person or pictures of my personal library. I have books everywhere. Shelves and shelves of books. I have learned to love books. It's books, books, and more books. I can't stop buying them either. I have books that are just in stacks waiting to be read and yet, I still end up buying another one that seems so fascinating.

The truth is, books changed my life. I couldn't have done what I've done without books. I would hate to admit this to my grade school teachers who begged me to read books as a child. I wasn't a fan of books as a kid. I did my best to avoid them.

Eventually I was fortunate to learn that there are so many experts that are willing to share their knowledge and experience and then they write it down and sell that valuable information for only $10 or $20 dollars. This information sometimes took decades for somebody to learn and accumulate and here I could buy it all summarized and read it in a few hours. How can you beat a deal like that?

Part of a health and wellness program is understanding all facets of health and wellness. This includes more than just physical health. It includes mental health, spiritual health, and emotional health. These are all related to one another.

For example, when you get worn down emotionally and stressed out, that impacts your physical health. You are more prone to have those emotional triggers influence what you eat, drink, what you do, and how you sleep. Again, things all come together full circle. We need to be healthy in all areas of the human existence.

Along with exercising your body, it's very important that you continuously exercise your mind. This does more than just prevent health issues like Alzheimer's or other cognitive issues. Exercising the mind keeps you sharp, allows you to grow, learn, and develop along your journey.

Today's topic is on the importance of exercising the mind through reading (or listening to) a good book of your choice. Now I'm not talking about "50 Shades of Gray" or "Harry Potter" for entertainment. I'm talking about a book that can help you learn more about some topic that relates to your health. It could be on nutrition, exercise, running, sleeping better, stress reduction, meditation, habit creation, or on a role model that demonstrates success to you.

The point is, books do a lot of good to the brain and in turn, do a lot of good that will then trickle down to your physical health, spiritual health, mental health, and overall health. These relate and integrate with one another.

"You can't buy happiness, but you can buy books and that's kind of the same thing." – Unknown

Your objective over the next few days is to goof around at the bookstore or on Amazon. Buy a book that tickles your brain and teaches you something new and exciting about the human body. Expand your mind and you'll experience more success over a lifetime. Pick a book that appeals to you and will be fun to read. Don't pick a complicated or boring textbook. Reading should be fun, enjoyable, and relaxing. It it's not, you are picking the wrong books to read or listen to.

Don't be afraid to explore audio books either if you spend a lot of time in the car or you want to walk and listen at the same time. That's a great way to kill two birds with one stone. Go for a walk and fill your brain with goodness.

What This Means To Me – And You
Progress will happen when you continuously accomplish the two steps of acquiring knowledge AND implementing that knowledge into your own life. Unless you act and implement the knowledge into your everyday life, nothing happens. There will be no results. There will be no personal breakthroughs or transformations.

There are a lot of people out there who are stuck in this endless pursuit of more knowledge, more books, more articles, and more learning courses. They seem to hope and believe that they will start doing something productive with all that knowledge, "once they have just a little bit more information to get started safely."

In similar fashion, there are many times where you have all the necessary knowledge to make a good health decision, but you will still choose poorly.

The principles of health success are not complicated items to understand. They are quite simple. In fact, understanding the principles is the simple part. Executing the principles daily for years on end is the hard part. Many people experience a lot of health failures, and all too often the health failures are self-inflicted.

BOOM! Easy-Peasy... Reading books is filling your brain with goodness and will allow you to reach your goals better and faster.

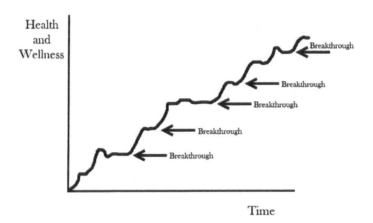

Day 9 – Hello Sunshine and Fresh Air!

Do you believe that doing healthy activities always has to be hard or seem like a sacrifice? Do you believe that positive benefits only come through struggle and painful exertion? What if I told you that this belief is completely wrong? Would it blow your mind?

Today's topic is something that is super easy-peasy but ignored by far too many people. It's the importance of getting outside in the sunshine and getting fresh air daily.

Now most people fall into traditional habits and behaviors in the developed world. They go to work and often spend all day indoors only to come home and hit the couch. But all that recycled air can have a whole host of negative impacts on your health. There are allergens, low oxygen levels, along with other indoor pollutants from things like carpeting, paint, or even cleaning products that are quite normal in indoor settings.

Getting outside for some sunshine and fresh air clears the lungs, provides fresh oxygen, and can lead to more energy and clarity of thoughts. This results in people feeling happier, healthier, and more energetic. HEY FREE ENERGY!!!

Natural sunlight is also important for obtaining your daily requirement of Vitamin D (something that most people are deficient in which leads to health consequences). Spending about 30 minutes a day can provide most people with their daily requirement of Vitamin D which is necessary for bone health, and reducing the risk of other diseases.

The combination of sunshine and fresh air has shown to reduce stress and depression. People that spend more time outside report feeling more relaxed afterwards. This leads to lower blood pressure and lower levels of cortisol (the stress hormone) but increases the amount of serotonin (the happy hormone) in the brain.

Increased exposure to sunshine is associated with decreased mental health distress. There is a direct correlation between those with mental health distress and reduced sun time hours.

Sunshine also impacts our sleep cycles as the sun assists in maintaining healthy melatonin production and a balanced body clock for sleep and wake cycles.

You may often feel time constrained like most people. It's like you just don't have enough hours in the day to do everything that you need to or want to do. That's where it helps when you start doing some things that **knock out multiple items at once**. Examples might include;

- You need sunshine and fresh air. What if you walk or run outside so that you not only are getting your sunshine and fresh air, but you are also knocking out your daily exercise goal? What if you listen to an audio book at the same time? Now you are REALLY becoming efficient with your time and following success principles.

- What if you went for a walk outside with your spouse or children? Now you are a positive influence on them, you encourage them to get some sunshine and fresh air and you both accumulate some walking steps that improve your circulation. You can talk and reconnect at the same time. Improved relationships lead to improved mental and spiritual health. Better mental and spiritual health leads to less stress and anxiety which leads to better physical health.

- Could you encourage a co-worker to discuss a project or company goal while walking outside for 15 minutes rather than chit-chatting at the water cooler or in a stuffy meeting room with no windows? Fresh air could help you think more clearly and eliminate some of the typical noise that is part of an office environment.

The essential point is that sunshine and fresh air are very important to get each day. Living in colder climates can make this a challenge which is why so many people in certain geographic areas experience Seasonal Affective Disorder (SAD) which is winter depression. But this makes sense because many people that live in colder climates may not get outdoors for months on end except to get the mail as quickly as possible or walk from the parking lot to the inside of the grocery store. That's just not enough exposure to sunshine or fresh air for a healthy life.

Are you getting enough sunshine and fresh air? Are you able to get in more steps outside while asking others to join you for social time or use that walk to fill your brain with goodness?

So today, tomorrow and the next day, get outside.

BOOM! Easy-Peasy... Getting a daily dose of sunshine and fresh air leads to improved health and happiness.

Self-Reliance

Hey, what's this, bonus reading? You thought the chapter was done! I wanted to sneak in a little extra material on the importance of being self-reliant and personal responsibility.

Health and wellness practitioners are very self-reliant, and take personal responsibility for their results. In fact, these two traits are common denominators amongst those who have accomplished successful health transformations.

Self-reliance does not mean that wellness practitioners can't or don't have political viewpoints. Nor does it mean that you can't believe in God, or think that luck isn't something that happens in life.

Plenty of wellness practitioners have political viewpoints. Plenty of healthy people believe in God. Plenty of healthy people believe in luck.

But while healthy people can believe in all those things, they also believe in themselves. They take a lot of personal responsibility for their outcomes in life.

Don't Play The Blame Game

If you are of the mindset that the reason you aren't where you think you should be in life is because of the government, your boss, your company, your friends, or your mommy, then it's doubtful you will find the self-tenacity to persevere in a lengthy process of achievement.

The biggest thing holding each of us back is often ourselves. Many life experiences could lead us astray in our journey and decision making. You may have grown up without a lot of money. You may not have had good role models. You may not have had good mentors. You may not have had the best public education growing up. You may not have had perfect parents. Your current job may stink. You may not have been given all the knowledge along the way that it takes to figure out this health improvement stuff. Add to that the fact that you may have a bunch of people around you that don't want to see you succeed.

Fair enough. Those could all be true and are very reasonable issues that would describe your obstacles. But it will take individual efforts to overcome those obstacles and succeed. Nobody else is going to do it for you. Nobody is going to figure out your exact circumstances and spoon feed what you need to do in a way that you could sit back, drink a beer, relax, and lose the muffin top around your waistband.

There are countless examples of individuals who encountered great obstacles in their life yet overcame them and still went on to accomplish their health goals and objectives. Some of these individuals grew up poor, in broken families, with little to no formal or quality education. Others had few financial resources at their disposal along the way. But they overcame their obstacles and pursued the goals that were important to them. You must find the courage to put out that same type of effort if you want to succeed.

In health and wellness, success comes as a function of the food you eat. You are 100% responsible for what goes in your mouth. Nobody forces food down your throat. Nobody forces you to stay up late watching TV. You must make those decisions for yourself. You must make those tradeoffs in life. That's part of the process.

Don't Wait For The Perfect Time

The best mindset is one where you just openly acknowledge that you have a multitude of issues that aren't ideal in your life right now. But you must realize they aren't going to get any better unless you do something for yourself to change the circumstances.

Maybe you will have to get new friends. Maybe you will need to learn new skills. Maybe you will need to develop entirely new habits. Maybe you will need to exercise. Maybe you will need to read some books or get a second job to pay for the courses that you need to take to acquire the necessary knowledge to get you unstuck from wherever you are in your process right now.

These potential changes can certainly appear to be overwhelming and scary. They are scary. You may get nervous and afraid. You are certainly not alone in your feelings. Change is scary. Change takes time. Change takes effort. The results don't normally start appearing overnight. That is ok. Plenty of others have made the journey and are happy that they overcame their fears and insecurities.

It is not practical or efficient to try and change every single item in your life all at once. What is important is that you select one or two items that are most important to your future success and get started on those items immediately. Start today.

It's ok. It's all right. Take a deep breath. Change is good. It's uncertain. Embrace the change. Get excited about the change. Change is an integral part of the process of achievement. To make progress means constant change and evolution. If you remain in a constant state of being, there is no progress. You must be willing to help yourself because if you are waiting around in the wrong places for something good to just hit you over the head, you are not likely to progress.

"A lot of people are waiting for their ship to come in. Too bad they are waiting at the bus stop."

Health

Principles

ARE YOU BUILDING MOMENTUM EACH DAY?

THE FOUNDATIONS OF HEALTH SUCCESS

- Eat healthy
- Exercise your body
- Exercise your mind
- Exposure to sunshine and fresh air
- Get adequate sleep and rest
- Reduce stress and anxiety
- Avoid harmful substances (toxins, chemicals, drugs, alcohol, additives, and preservatives in foods.)

Day 10 – Getting Adequate Sleep

What if there was a component of weight loss and health success that had little to do with diet and exercise but is most often ignored? Would you want to add that missing ingredient?

Are you like most people who wake up tired day after day? You have no energy, are lethargic, and feel drowsy? You can't think straight. You don't want to do anything physical outside of work. You feel as though you are walking around like a zombie day after day needing caffeine, sugar, or energy drinks to carry you as you crash and burn every few hours.

Most people dread that alarm going off each morning. They lie in bed and think to themselves, "Oh brother, here we go again..."

You would think being so tired would make people want to get more sleep. That would make sense, wouldn't it? Are you like most people who aren't getting adequate sleep?

Poor sleeping habits have a wide variety of negative impacts on your life. Lack of sleep leads to diminished cognitive performance (that means you can't think straight!) Lack of sleep means lack of health.

Sleep regulates your hormones, allows your body to repair itself, and allows your body to rejuvenate itself. Fat loss becomes much more difficult without adequate sleep!

Today is about the importance of getting 8 hours of sleep each night and having regular sleeping habits. If you can follow a regular sleep schedule, you can live a happier and healthier life. It's important to be consistent in your sleep patterns. Pick a time to go to bed and pick a time to get out of bed each morning. Make sure that it allows you to get 8 hours of sleep between those two times.

Your body has an internal clock. It's called a circadian rhythm (body clock). You want to allow your body clock to start functioning as intended. Give yourself every chance at success.

Sleep has a sneaky way of impacting your weight loss and health pursuits. It takes emotional and mental fortitude to make good choices in life. How many times have you experienced a sequence of events such as the following;

- You didn't get enough sleep and are very tired for a day or two afterwards.
- You just can't think straight. It's like your brain is in a fog.
- You are more irritable and cranky than normal. Small things start to trigger bigger feelings and emotions.
- It's hard to keep a positive attitude and stay motivated when worn down and tired.

- You skip a workout or exercise – too tired!
- You argue with a loved one – too cranky!
- You lose motivation – too mentally weak!
- Life starts to beat you down and you become discouraged. You can't keep a positive mental attitude. You start to believe that everything is just too hard.
- You seek comfort and immediate gratification. You need something that can make you feel good and quick. You end up eating junk food, an unhealthy meal, drink non-healthy drinks, and go severely backwards in your pursuit of health and fitness.
- It all started because you let yourself get worn down and tired due to a lack of sleep.

Once you realize how health principles impact one another, you can start achieving higher levels of success with far less effort. You need to be strong physically, mentally, and emotionally.

This occurs much easier when you are recovered and rested and ready to knock the ball out of the park the next day rather than dragging your butt around. Accomplishing goals starts to become automatic and without much effort at all. It's like there is no longer any resistance in your life.

Give yourself a chance to win at this process in the easiest way possible. One way to expedite your results is by doing something that your body is already telling you to do – get more sleep and do it on a regular schedule.

That may mean going to bed at 10:00pm and waking up at 6:00am. Or 11:00pm and 7:00am. Or 9:00pm and 5:00am. You get to pick what works for you. Just start going to bed at the same time (and probably earlier than you normally do).

Pay attention to the details that may impact the quality of your sleep as well;

- The quality of your sheets and mattress (are you sleeping on a piece of junk with newspapers as sheets?)
- The temperature of your bedroom at night (should be cool, not hot)
- Is the room dark?
- Did you consume caffeine and sugar within a few hours of going to bed?
- Did you consume any foods that can be disruptive to sleep? An example would be chocolate which has theobromine in it. Theobromine is the compound that makes chocolate dangerous to pets. It increases heart rate and causes sleeplessness and could stay in the system for upwards of 12 to 24 hours. That means eating chocolate at lunch may still impact a person's sleep that night.
- Are you going to bed at different times and not allowing your body to get into a rhythm?
- Are you stressed and anxious and mentally consumed with things that are bothering you in life?
- Are you in poor physical condition with aches and pains that don't allow you to get comfortable at night?

- Are you taking prescription medications like beta blockers, alpha blockers, and/or antidepressants?

What you are learning is that health creates a lot of "what comes first, the chicken or the egg" scenarios. If you aren't healthy, it's hard to get quality sleep. If you aren't getting quality sleep, it's extremely hard to get and stay healthy.

BOOM! Easy-Peasy... Getting adequate sleep leads to improved health and happiness. Who would have thought that you could gain so many health and wellness benefits from just lying there dreaming about your health transformation?

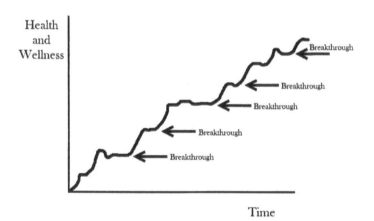

Daily Check-In

HOW DID YOU DO TODAY WITH YOUR GOALS?

- Are you building momentum and tracking results?
- Are you slowly substituting and crowding out bad foods with less bad foods and maybe even the good foods listed in the table on page 71?
- Are you getting daily exercise consistently? (Don't worry about the workload just yet.)
- Are you acquiring knowledge and implementing it?
- Did you get any sunshine and fresh air today?
- Did you get in 8 hours of sleep last night and are you setting yourself up to get 8 hours of sleep tonight?

Day 11 – Take a Breath

Losing weight, becoming healthy and feeling wonderful is sometimes a bit more physiologically complicated than most people realize. That's certainly not to say it's impossible. Plenty of people have learned how to live a healthy lifestyle with excellent fitness and enjoy an energetic body that feels years younger than its calendar based age.

But losing weight and being fit isn't just about calorie restriction. Did you know that stress can cause weight gain and impair your physical, mental, and emotional health?

Stress can come in many forms. It could be stemming from work, or debts, or relationships, or even poor health itself. That chronic stress plays a big role in weight gain and weight loss prevention making it much harder for you to accomplish your health goals. Stress leads to more mental anxiety and it becomes a hard trap to escape from.

Research shows that when people are stressed, they are much more apt to eat more and drink more (as in bad stuff like alcohol, not good ole' H2O!) You may have experienced this yourself. How many times have you come home from a hard day of work at wits end and try to relieve some of that pent-up frustration through food and drink (or worse!)

Your body has a stress hormone called cortisol and cortisol rises during stressful events. Elevated cortisol levels can impact your insulin levels which regulates your blood sugar levels. This in turn can trigger cravings for sugary and fatty foods (the exact foods that you are trying to avoid.)

That's why people will reach for a beer, a hard drink, a cigarette, a bowl of ice cream, or a bag of chips rather than an apple or some cut up veggies when they are under a lot of stress.

Understanding this link alone will give you a significant leg up in your quest for health. It will allow you to stop, take a step back, and ask yourself, "Am I really hungry, or am I just stressed out?" There are things to do when you find yourself stressed out and one of the easiest and most powerful ones is to just stop and breathe.

When I say stop and breathe, I mean you are really going to stop and breathe and breathe **BIG**! You should use this powerful technique whenever anything upsetting happens and **BEFORE** you react or respond to whatever is causing the stress.

4-7-8 Breath Technique

You are going to do what is called the 4-7-8 Breath Technique. It is a proven way to successfully help the body respond to stress. It is super simple and can be done at any time and as often as you want. It should be done twice a day as a regular habit. There is plenty of information about this technique on the internet. Here is what you need to get started in order to enjoy the benefits of this proven technique right away;

- Place and keep the tip of your tongue against the top of your front teeth where the gum and teeth come together.
- Exhale firmly and completely through your mouth.
- Close your mouth and inhale through your nose for 4 seconds.
- Hold your breath for 7 seconds.
- Exhale completely through your mouth for 8 seconds.
- This sequence counts as 1 full breath. Repeat this sequence for a total of 4 breaths.

A good part of living a life of health and wellness is learning to simplify your life and diminish the amount of stress that you expose yourself to. Getting your cortisol levels to come down is a great place to start. This will take time, but the journey is well worth it.

A happy life is one where things all start coming together at once for you. Your health will improve. Your relationships will improve. Your personal finances will improve. Stress comes down. Your free time goes up. Your knowledge and wisdom increase. Success principles become automatic and require little if any thought whatsoever.

These success items happen a little bit at a time. It all builds through the power of "M." It makes no difference where you start. It only matters where you end up.

If you are a smart phone user and love using apps, there are several breathing apps available to use as well. You may find these helpful and valuable when working on your breathing.

So today, tomorrow, and the next day, stop a few times and do some 4-7-8's.

BOOM! Easy-Peasy... Learning how to control your stress and control your anxiety through breathing techniques like the 4-7-8 method can absolutely lead to improved health and happiness. All you must do is breathe and chill out for a few seconds to reset the systems.

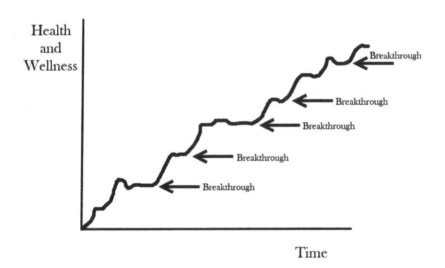

Day 12 –Crowd Out And Substitute

Awesome Health Isn't Random

You will come across many individuals who believe that healthy and energetic people are just lucky in life. They believe that superior health was handed out randomly (or genetically), as if people were just blindly selected from a giant list.

Many people graduate from college, find jobs in corporate America, and then eventually expect to be hand-picked to become a success in all areas of life. These people end up extremely disappointed and confused. When their health starts to diminish they can become frustrated, stressed, hopeless, or jealous.

Healthy people don't put their faith in the luck of the draw or get stuck in a fixed mindset believing that there is nothing that could be done to change their physical qualities. They do put themselves in favorable positions that increase the odds of success, but they work hard at evolving, adapting, and learning as they proceed towards their goals.

No Invitation Needed

The good news about joining the ranks of the healthy is that you never have to wait for an invitation to jump on the wellness bandwagon. It is open to all who complete the process of achievement, live by health principles, and do the work necessary. It is non-discriminating. The healthy club has no race quotas. The healthy club does not care what sex you are, what religion you practice, what language you speak, or what political party you tend to favor.

The healthy club only cares if you can learn and implement the principles of health into your daily lives on a consistent basis. The healthy club will allow you to stay a member so long as you can live by the principles of health throughout your entire journey. Old age will eventually set in, but you can greatly extend the **quality** of all those years in-between now and then.

The principles of health success are universal and could be applied in any period of time, in any geography around the world. Health knows no boundaries. Anybody can join the club.

Turning The Ship On Bad Habits and Behaviors
Before I finally figured out the path to health and wellness, I had a big problem. I couldn't stop eating certain foods and drinking certain beverages. To make matters worse, once I started eating or drinking those foods and beverages, it was like a switch went off inside of me.

I literally could not stop eating and drinking until it felt like I was ready to explode. Then it would sink in as to what I did to myself and I would feel so devastated. I'd feel like a complete failure. The satisfaction from the food would wear off and I'd feel terrible in many ways.

Here I was dreaming (and praying) that somehow, I was going to finally lose the weight and start feeling better about myself. I would dream of wearing clothes that fit me better. I would dream of having more energy. I would dream of just being happier with myself. Yet, when the decisive moment would appear, I'd crumble like a coffee cake that was being lifted to my mouth.

Then I would have to start all over again, dreaming that tomorrow would be different. That somehow tomorrow I would be able to fix all my eating habits with the snap of a finger. That somehow, I magically would turn into a different person overnight.

That magic never happened. I never changed miraculously overnight. But I did change…slowly…and built momentum.

When I would feel tired, angry, stressed, hungry, anxious, or even just bad about myself, I would seek out ways to make myself feel better. I'd use food and drinks to do that back then. Perhaps you could relate to this. I justified these actions by telling myself that I deserved it because I was having a rough day or that I needed a distraction from my problems.

But it turned out, my problems were only being compounded by the choices I was making when trying to alleviate the bad feelings and pain I was having related to my problems. It was like a vicious circle of health doom.

Something had to give. I just kept going on and on like that. It was starting to become exhausting. I finally had enough.

But rather than continuously trying to change everything overnight, I tried a different approach and it led to significant and lasting success. I broke the issue down into two distinct components;

1. Recognize when I am having a "triggering moment." I had to first recognize when I was eating not to feed myself required nutrients, but rather feeding myself to dull some other pain, emotion, or feeling. I was eating too much for comfort and pleasure to cover something else up. That had to change.

2. When I did stop and ask myself, "Why are you desiring food right now?" I WOULDN'T prevent myself from eating necessarily. That's what I tried repeatedly in the past and it clearly wasn't working. I just kept failing when I tried to stop eating cold turkey. Rather, I started using a technique of "**crowding out and substitution.**"

Crowding out and substitution allowed me to use the principles of consistency and "M" (that good old momentum principle). But here is the catch, I would make sure I was pro-actively PREPARED for such an occasion. I'd be ready to go with alternatives to the foods I was drawn to in the past.

I was committed to slowly changing my habits in a way that led to lasting success. When I found myself stressed and normally reaching for some potato chips and a sugared soft-drink, I'd have some salted sweet potato chips and some iced-tea ready to crowd out the bad. I'd allow myself to eat while taking note of my emotional state.

The salt from the sweet potato chips would make me thirsty. The iced tea would quench my thirst. Soon enough, I'd be stuffed to the gills. But rather than loading up on regular potato chips and carbonated sugar, I found a way to crowd out the bad and move towards something that was "less bad."

After a while, I moved away from salted sweet potato chips and towards salted nuts. Sugared iced-tea eventually moved towards unsweetened or low-calorie tea or flavored water.

Over time, I would find myself hungry during the day and maybe even stressed but I lost the desire for fatty fried snacks, or racks of ribs, or carbonated sugar (which was my hardest habit to break by far!) I'd be grateful for a super sweet sumo mandarin orange or an apple with almond butter. I know that sounds crazy, but it is true. It just took a while, but it worked for the long-term.

You see, I learned that we have a bunch of pre-programmed automated mental habits that we run for ourselves in our brains without even thinking about them. Some other triggers usually initiate these habits. The triggers could be any host of stressors or events in our lives. I had to recognize those triggers while they were happening in real time to break those loops.

Imagine drawing a straight line from the top of a piece of paper to the bottom creating two columns. On the left were the worst foods and drinks that I was eating and drinking. On the right were the healthiest foods and drinks I should be eating and drinking.

Bad Foods I Was Eating	Best Foods I Should Be Eating

I found myself failing repeatedly when I would try and move my eating and drinking habits all the way from the left to all the way on the right overnight. It was just one short-term attempt after another that ended in failure. It wasn't until I just tried to move the needle bit by bit by using the crowding out and substitution technique that I started making lasting progress. I just never wanted to go backwards.

I no longer tried to substitute pizza for broccoli. I couldn't sustain that after a week or two. I'd quit. It was too hard, too scary, and too painful. It also ended repeatedly in complete failure.

But I would try eating pizza without sausage and pepperoni. Then pizza without meat and with a single thing that might even be considered healthy (like a vegetable topping). Maybe an olive or a mushroom on it. Then I would substitute normal dough for gluten free dough. Then maybe chicken fingers rather than pizza. Then chicken fingers that were air-fried or baked rather than deep fried.

There are million ways a person can use crowding out and substitution. The key is to just think this through and start implementing it in your daily life. What is one thing that you could do to crowd out something bad from your diet and substitute it with something "less bad."

If you can just keep going with this exercise, one day you are going to wake up just like me on the right side of the page. You'll be eating all kinds of good stuff and having absolutely no desire to fill your belly with bad stuff. You will have achieved long-term success, but you took it slower which made it more sustainable. You gave your body ample time to slowly adapt at a reasonable pace.

What you are learning throughout this daily process is that if something is sustainable, it will be more consistent. If something can be done consistently, then the success principle of "M" can be applied. "M" is the all-powerful principle of momentum. **All goodness can be built with "M."** Allow your body the time to adapt.

To think that you are going to eat perfect for the rest of your days with the snap of a finger may be a strategy that keeps failing you just like it failed me. It wasn't until I took the long-road approach and just kept crowding out and substituting the bad with the "less bad" that the magic finally started to happen.

Days turned into weeks, weeks into months, and months into years.

Somehow, I woke up with six-pack abs and my dreams finally came true.

Today, tomorrow, and the next day, stop a few times and do some crowding out and substituting choosing "less bad" foods in place of "bad foods." It's super easy-peasy this way. All you must do is try and not to go backwards once you begin. You can do it this way and it is sustainable.

Day 13 – Morning Rocket Fuel

It would be obvious to say that eating healthy is essential for long-term health and wellness. Not to mention that eating healthy expedites our success on losing weight, looking good, and feeling fantastic about ourselves.

But I found that eating healthy isn't as simple as knowing or being told to eat healthy foods like vegetables. Sure, eating vegetables is an absolute requirement for long-term health, but what is a person to do when they are just getting started on this journey of health and may hate vegetables like I did when I started? I hated vegetables and many other healthy foods and went out of my way to avoid them.

Once I finally concluded that trying to completely change my life all at once and turn my life upside down was too much of a shock to my system, I knew I needed a different approach. I started making changes focusing only on one meal at a time. I picked breakfast.

Focusing on breakfast did a few things that ended up working well for me. First, it obviously is the first meal of the day. If I could make small changes to that first meal and become consistent, that would not only allow me to build momentum "M," but I'd feel good and confident in myself for the remainder of that day. I would get a win for myself right off the bat and carry that victory for the rest of the day. I could at least go to bed each night knowing I made progress.

The second thing that worked well for me was that I had the most focus the first thing in the morning to make positive improvements. The day had yet to kick my ass, get me down, beat me up, and spit me out. I didn't need food or drinks in the morning to help me get through any emotional triggers because the day didn't even start yet. I had that going in my favor.

Now today, I could tell you that I have a fruit and vegetable smoothie with all kinds of extra super foods in it that would probably blow your mind or may even intimidate you. That's not the important thing to recognize right now. The important thing is to just remind you that small incremental improvements that are sustainable is the most important thing.

If the small changes are sustainable, you will be consistent. If you are consistent, you can build "M" and with momentum, you can do anything over a long stretch of time. The success will be permanent and long lasting. Nothing will be just a fad for you. You won't fade-out, flame-out, and fail-out. You will win!

The other thing to note on this item and other health related matters is that there is always some way to improve something. It may get to be super small, but improvements never stop. There is always something that could be improved upon.

It's like we talked about in yesterday's chapter, imagine a line on a sheet of paper that splits the page into two columns. On the left is the worst possible breakfast you could eat as far as human nutrition goes. Maybe it is chocolate covered donuts fried in bacon grease with cheese and crystal meth sprinkled on top. One the right is my Rocket Fuel Smoothie which we'll talk about later in this process.

I'm more than happy to share the recipe for my rocket fuel smoothie but quite frankly, your body can't handle that just yet. Just like my body can no longer handle chocolate donuts. If I ate Fruit Loops or chocolate donuts, I would be vomiting within the hour and would have massive stomach pains. My body no longer craves nor tolerates that kind of garbage in my system.

But it took a while to transform myself. You see, the body is **ADAPTIVE**. That's very important to understand. The body can change over time and adapt to different things and environments. You are learning how to harness this adaptive power of the human body.

You have your line on the sheet of paper. Don't try and go all the way from the left side to all the way over to the right side over night or in a week or even a month. This is going to take some time to allow your body to develop new habits and cravings and nutritional requirements. Allow your body to ADAPT.

If you do this right, your body will start craving what is good for it and will start rebelling and protesting the consumption of things that are bad for it. It happened to me and it will happen to you.

For the time being, just put a lot of emphasis on changing your breakfast as your primary focus. If you can make changes in your lunch, dinner, and snacks along the way and you are super motivated, that's great, but don't rush things at the expense of messing up your progress on your breakfast.

You want to start the day on the right foot, make some changes, bank some wins, and then head into your day knowing that you made progress on lasting goals that are going to lead to long-term success.

It will help you if you write down what you are currently eating so over time, you can make sure you are progressing and making incremental changes for the better. Sustainable, consistent progress building on "M."

So today, tomorrow and the next day, let's just start crowding out and substituting items on your breakfast. It's super easy-peasy this way. All you must do is try and not go backwards with your progress. You can do it this way and it is sustainable. Keep up the good work. You are changing from the inside out.

Day 14 – Just A Tiny Bit More Than Yesterday

Many people dream of becoming an overnight success and dropping weight lightning fast. They seek immediate results and look for short-cuts to success. In their attempts to speed things up, they usually end up slowing things down or failing all together.

On Day 7 of Easy-Peasy health and wellness, I gave you the "Daily Exercise Secret." I told you why people fail at sticking to an exercise program even if they have the best intentions in the world. They have the same resolutions each year, but then they flame out big time. They flop, they stop, and they quit.

I told you that these people that come out like gangbusters are doomed from the start because they aren't using the **principle of "M."** They don't start out with something that is sustainable based on where their body is at that moment in time. Rather, they started out where they thought they should be or where they dreamed about being. Unfortunately for them, it just doesn't work that way.

I gave you the two critical components for an outstanding exercise program. They are:

1. Consistency
2. Workload (the volume and intensity of your workouts)

The most important component is the first one and that is consistency. Consistency must come first. It's far more important than workload at the early stages when changing your daily routines.

If you recall, we talked about Michael Phelps in how he used the power of "M" to become the most decorated Olympic athlete of all time. He was consistent like no other while he built up his workload over two decades.

Fortunately, you don't have to be Michael Phelps, nor do you have to train like him to get the health and wellness results that you desire. You only need to do what is necessary to live a life of health and wellness.

Day 7 was about starting small. It doesn't matter how small you start because as "M" kicks in over your lifetime, the results are going to come soon enough and will be amazing in time. But the results you desire can't come if you don't start and stay consistent with a sustainable workload.

Starting small could have meant any of the following even if they seem ridiculously easy;

- 1 pushup
- 1 sit-up
- 1 lunge
- 1 pull-up
- 1 squat with your own body weight
- 1 game of basketball

- 1 dance in your living room to good music
- walking steps beyond your normal routine (intentional additional steps beyond the mailbox, or intentionally parking further away from your office building or grocery store.)

People often state, "What's the point of doing so little?" You see, it doesn't matter how small you start. That's the beauty of "M." What matters more than anything is that you just start with intentional exercise and start working that into your daily routine and build consistency habits.

And guess what happens? If you did start on Day 7 with 1 pushup, or 1 sit-up, or 1 two-minute dance, a week has now gone by (Yes, time flies by one way or another.) And now one week later, guess what your body is now able to do easily? It's probably anxious and ready to do 2 push-ups, or 2 sit-ups, or dance for 4 minutes, or walk for 10 minutes straight **WITHOUT FEELING OVER-STRAINED!**

I can't stress enough how important it is to only do what is **sustainable** for the rest of your life. Don't do any more than that or you will just flame out, flop out, and stop like all the other dreamers out there. If you can easily do 5 push-ups, then do 5 push-ups. But do them daily. If you can walk 5,000 steps in your current daily routine right now, then walk 5,000 steps daily.

Now if you can do 5 pushups a day sustainably and one day you get this crazy idea that leads you to push yourself unrealistically and you try to max out and do 10 pushups, what's going to happen this early in your program? You are going to be so sore from doing twice what you should have done that the next day you can't even do 5 push-ups. That means you must skip a day of exercise. That means you are no longer consistent. That means you weren't sticking to what is sustainable. That means you aren't using the power of "M."

This is about doing **sustainable exercise consistently** utilizing the power of "M." You are developing lifelong habits first that will provide the foundation for increasing the workload over time. As you know, the time flies by anyways, so let that work in your favor.

What's Holding You Back?

The world is now a two-edge sword. On one hand we have never had access to as much knowledge and information as we do now, especially with the power of the internet and the ease of access to books, podcasts, articles, blogs, and television. On the other hand, we have never had more distractions and noise pollution in our head as to what are the core elements of success in a health and wellness lifestyle.

Your success or failure should not be due to the lack of resources or information. Instead, it's due to a lack of core principles, coupled with a significant lack of the implementation of those principles. Health and wellness is a lifestyle choice and a way of life in and of itself. You must choose whether you want to live your life in that fashion. You must choose to apply the tools and information that you have access to in this wired, globally connected world we live in.

The Starting Point

It doesn't matter what your desired destination is. That is for you to decide what is appropriate for yourself. But regardless of your eventual desires, everyone has a starting point on their health and wellness journey. Don't get distracted based on where you are starting. Many people must hit rock bottom and must experience terrible health before they realize their internal desires and values. Focus on where you want to be in the future.

Each day, you start over again with your health, either improving or diminishing. You will have a starting point, and for health and wellness practitioners, they know that each day is a brand new starting point.

Many people believe that their health is a fixed item programmed entirely by genetics and that there is nothing that they could do to change their situation. But that is simply not true. There are thousands of examples of people who have completely transformed themselves from one physical being into another.

We've seen people lose hundreds of pounds, become a marathon runner, take up martial arts or some other sport, or just learn how to live a healthy, happy, and active life where their physical abilities allow them to participate in all kinds of fun activities that the world has to offer.

So today, tomorrow, and the next day, let's just keep a daily exercise program going no matter how small or insignificant it may seem right now. It's super easy-peasy this way. All you must do is try and not go backwards. When you do it this way, it is sustainable. Keep up the good work. You are changing yourself and transforming yourself from the inside out.

Day 15 – Listen Up! Here's An Easy Tip For Improvement

If you are like me, you probably feel like there just isn't enough time in the day to do everything that you need to get done and want to get done. It feels like you are on a treadmill and somebody is sneaking up beside you and cranking up the speed – FASTER! FASTER! FASTER!

That's why it is so important to multi-task on items that can be combined. It allows you to accomplish two, three, or maybe even four objectives at once. If you go back to core life principles of success, you probably have figured out a few things for yourself at this point;

- If a person's finances are a mess, they probably are going to live a hard life.
- If a person's health is a mess, they probably are going to live a hard life.
- If a person has bad relationships, they probably are going to live a hard life.
- If a person has poor time management skills, they probably are going to live a hard life.
- If a person can't do things that make them happy and fulfilled over the long-term, they probably are going to live a hard life.

Magic happens when you can do tasks that knock out items from multiple success principles. For example, what if you liked playing basketball and after work one day were able to shoot hoops with some friends. What would that activity do for you? Well;

- Playing hoops is usually free, so that is helping your finances and preventing you from spending money. Finances…check!
- Playing hoops counts as exercise and improves your health. Health…check!
- Playing hoops with friends is a great social activity. You will build bonds, laugh, and keep friendships going. Relationships…check!
- Playing hoops can be done in an hour or so and is close to the house (maybe even in your own driveway). Time management…check!
- Playing hoops is fun. Fun and laughter makes people happy. Happiness…check!

But enough about hoops. I really want to encourage you to learn how to multi-task with your health and happiness activities. We are all crunched for time. We are all running around like crazy (and not running in a good way).

When you learn how to multi-task on key principles of health and wellness, great things happen, and your happiness is sure to escalate.

Look for ways to accomplish multiple principles with one activity. Be smart with your time. Don't waste one of your most precious assets. We all have the same 24 hours in a day and 168 hours in a week. How you use that precious time is the difference between a hard life and a great life.

Listen UP

Another example of using your time more efficiently is by listening to podcasts or audio books while doing other mundane tasks to gain valuable knowledge and exercise your brain.

PODCASTS?!?!? Are you still one of those people that ask, "What's a podcast?" It's simply a digital audio file made available on the internet for downloading to a computer or mobile device like your phone. Most phones now have apps for downloading, organizing, and listening to podcasts.

I can honestly say that podcasts have changed my life. I barely listen to normal or satellite radio anymore because I've been addicted to various podcasts. My only regret is that I didn't start listening to podcasts years ago. They are that powerful and useful.

Podcasts allow you to listen to some of the most fun, entertaining, educational, and inspirational information FOR FREE! (Great on the budget!) If your car has Bluetooth capabilities, you can play your podcasts over your phone and have it come out your speakers in your car. You can listen with headphones while walking around the block. You can listen on lunch breaks, driving to and from work, on long trips, in the evenings while lying in bed, or even while soaking in a tub.

I even bought a portable Bluetooth speaker, so I could listen to podcasts while working in the kitchen preparing meals or playing with my dogs in the backyard.

There are literally thousands of various podcast series out there. There is something for everyone. But I recommend that you find, listen, and follow the ones that resonate personally with you regarding your health, wellness, and fitness. This allows you to spice up tedious commutes, cut the grass, do laundry, cook meals, get through workouts, all by just pushing "play" on your smart phone. Sound too good to be true? It isn't. Podcasts are wonderful.

My favorites for health include the Rich Roll Podcast, Ben Greenfield's podcast, or the Strenuous Life podcast (which has a jiu-jitsu theme to it). But maybe you will like the Fat-Burning Man Show or Spartan Up (hosted by the guy who created the Spartan Race Series). There are so many to choose from and there is something for everybody. Find a few that work for you.

Listening to podcasts is one of the most entertaining and easy ways to increase knowledge, gather information, and stay motivated on your quest for personal improvement. The best part of it is that listening to them is so EASY-PEASY.

An Easy Way To Consume More Books

The same is true for audio books. Many people don't have the time to sit and read physical books each day and exercise their brain in a stimulating way. Audio books are a solution to this problem. As physical book sales are declining, audio books are thriving. You can listen to audio books in the same way you could listen to podcasts.

Use your time efficiently. Instead of commuting to work each day listening to the same crap news or same music that you have heard a hundred times, get into the habit of listening to books and accumulating more knowledge.

So today, tomorrow, and the next day, start building your brain by listening to podcasts and audio books. It's super easy-peasy this way. All you must do is try and not go backwards. You can do it this way and it is sustainable. Keep up the good work. You are changing yourself and transforming yourself from the inside out.

Health Principles

ARE YOU BUILDING MOMENTUM EACH DAY?

THE FOUNDATIONS OF HEALTH SUCCESS

- Eat healthy
- Exercise your body
- Exercise your mind
- Exposure to sunshine and fresh air
- Get adequate sleep and rest
- Reduce stress and anxiety
- Avoid harmful substances (toxins, chemicals, drugs, alcohol, additives, and preservatives in foods.)

Day 16 – Halfway Home Review

Can you believe that you are halfway through your 30-day cycle of Easy-Peasy Health and Wellness?   What I wanted to do with this chapter is just take a time out and review what you have covered to assist in absorbing and implementing the new knowledge. Repetition is critically important on any learning endeavor.

In addition, you are learning to understand why so many people fail at their health and wellness objectives. They move their focus away from proven principles and forget about what matters. They do this even if doing what matters is easier to do than they realize if they stick to what is reasonable for themselves.

What's Your "WHY?"

This is a great time for reflection to just remind yourself on your "why." Why is it important that you improve your health, get more fit, and lose weight? Why are you willing to make personal changes now in your life? Why do you feel more motivated now to feel better about yourself than in the past? If you know deep down the answers to these important questions, you can stay focused on your "why" and you can stay the course, work through the obstacles, and achieve the personal success that you deserve.

Knowledge and Information – The "WHAT"

Next up on your journey to health and wellness is obtaining the knowledge and information that tells you "what" to do. This knowledge and information is helpful as it guides you on doing more of what we know works and doing less of what doesn't work. Part of this process is acknowledging that what you were doing in the past is in fact not providing you the results that you seek deep down.

Acknowledging your past is important to come to grips with because if you keep doing the same things as in the past, you would keep getting the same results that you got in the past. But you don't want those old results. You want new results. New results require new things to do. That's why the knowledge and information is important, so you learn "what" to do and "what not" to do.

Proven Principles

We already know what works in health and wellness. It's no mystery. There are common denominators to success and if you model yourself off these proven principles, you will find positive improvement in your own life.

Principles are timeless and your ability to implement the principles will mean the difference between success and failure. The most important principles for your health and wellness are:

1. **Eating healthy – what to eat, what not to eat**
2. **Exercise the body**
3. **Exercise the mind**
4. **Sunshine and fresh air**

5. **Adequate sleep, rest, and recovery**
6. **Reduce stress**
7. **Avoiding harmful substances**

You will notice that the 30-day Easy-Peasy process deals with implementing the principles of success. Mastery of the principles will take time. But the good news is that you are now working a program that leads to **lasting and permanent success**. This isn't about a fad diet or short-term trend. This is a success program that is about building a lasting lifestyle of winning the health battle that will reward you until your natural end of days due to aging.

As you work towards implementing the success principles, you are taking an approach that will work over the long-term. That means you aren't trying to turn your entire life upside down and shock your system in any way that is unsustainable.

Sustainable and Consistent Actions

Everything that you will be working on now and in the future, must be **sustainable**. If you are making small improvements that are **sustainable**, you will be able to implement those changes **consistently**. Anything that is done **consistently** will eventually turn into **habit**. Habits are powerful because once something is a habit, you can do it automatically with zero thought or effort. It becomes mindless and without resistance.

A Habit Of Success

Habits work both ways because you can implement good habits or bad habits. What you do for most of your waking hours is done on auto-pilot through habits. You wake up and start doing the exact same things repeatedly without even thinking about them. Replacing bad habits with good habits is essential for success in any endeavor.

Adaptive Bodies and Minds

Implementing good habits is possible because the human body is **ADAPTIVE**. The human body **adjusts and adapts** to most things that it is exposed to **repetitively**. That's why Eskimo's can live in cold climates, drug addicts can keep doing drugs, or why somebody else needs to run 10 miles a day to feel at peace with themselves. The body adapts to what it learns to do through **habits**. Your goal is to make your body adapt to positive changes and away from negative influences and behaviors.

The Power of "M"

By doing things that are **sustainable** you will build **consistency**. **Consistency** leads to **habits**. **Consistency** allows you to make small never-ending improvements that build "**M**." "**M**" **is the secret sauce**. Momentum is the magic that makes everything happen because with "M" anything is possible. Small 1% improvements add up to huge changes over time. Every breakthrough in human performance happens through "M." "M" can't happen without good **habits** that are built upon **consistency**.

You Have To Believe It To Achieve It

Finally, success requires the support of your internal belief system. You must believe you can change. You must visualize yourself living a happy life as a healthy person. You may not know exactly how good it feels to be healthy, fit, and energetic right now, but you must have faith that it is SOOO much better than being unhealthy, lethargic, and on track for all kinds of chronic diseases. You must believe it to achieve it.

The first 30 days focus entirely on the "what" portion of health and fitness. It is acquiring the core knowledge and understanding of how you are building a new life supported by proven principles of health and fitness. That foundation will allow you to build upwards from there. It's no different than building a big and strong pyramid. You can't build up and live a life of your dreams without a strong base and foundation.

It's all coming together. Keep up the good work. You probably don't even realize how much progress you are making mentally, physically, and emotionally proceeding through this journey because it is so Easy-Peasy! That's the beauty of this method. You aren't trying to change everything in your life all at once, but you are putting all the pieces in place to completely transform yourself from the inside-out that will result in a lifetime of achievement.

Daily Check-In

ARE YOU BUILDING MOMENTUM EACH DAY?

HOW DID YOU DO TODAY WITH YOUR GOALS?

- Did you track any results?
- Did you eat some healthy foods?
- Did you get some exercise?
- Did you get any sunshine and fresh air?
- Did you get adequate sleep last night?
- Did you stop and take in some deep breaths?
- Did you start out your day with a rocket fuel breakfast?
- Did you listen to or read anything to enhance your learning?

Day 17 – Bye-Bye Blue Lights

One of the core principles of health and wellness is getting adequate sleep, rest, and recovery. When you are well rested, you have the energy to take on the world and accomplish your dreams. Most people require 8 hours of quality sleep to fully recharge the batteries and allow your body to rebuild itself from the daily breakdown that cells and physiological systems experience.

Did you know that blue lights can impact the quality of your sleep? Blue light is short-wavelength-enriched light that is emitted from most electronic devices like smart phones, televisions, tablet computers, and desktop computers.

Blue light affects levels of the sleep hormone melatonin more than other light wavelengths. Once your melatonin levels are impacted, your sleep can be disturbed and disrupted as your natural body clock (circadian rhythm) is shifted.

The latest research shows that once our circadian clocks are altered, bad health effects can result. With a circadian rhythm that is off, you will sleep less hours and with a lack of quality (deep) sleep. A lack of sleep quantity along with poor quality impacts other hormonal functions. When you don't sleep well, that means you are tired and worn down the next day. When you are tired and worn down the next day, it's much easier (and attractive) to skip workouts, make poor eating choices, become stressed, and become unraveled. This can lead to further mental weakness and sickness all the way to clinical depression.

Ask yourself this, "Are you more or less patient with life when you are tired or well rested?" Yeah, I thought so!

Your sleep is a critical component to your health, wellness, and weight loss program. There are a few things you can do to help you get your beauty sleep. One of the big ones is to reduce your exposure to blue light sources in the evening hours. How can you do that? Here are some good starting points;

- Turn off electronic devices at least an hour or two before you are scheduled to go to bed/sleep at night.
- Read a paper book or listen to a podcast, or relaxing music, rather than watching TV, surfing social media, or reading an electronic reader prior to bed.
- Many electronic devices now have a "night-shift" mode which changes the color on your screens to warmer tones with less blue light. Explore these setting on your phone or tablet computers.
- Wear blue light blocking glasses in the evening if you want to watch TV all the way up to your scheduled bedtime. I have multiple pairs of blue light blocking glasses that I purchased through Swanwick Sleep found at www.swanwicksleep.com

If you want to supercharge your fat burning and energy levels, you need to be hitting on all cylinders. That means running the gamut on all the principles of health success. Give yourself every chance to succeed by getting a good night's sleep and that starts by reducing and eliminating blue light sources one to two hours prior to going to bed.

Keeping Yourself Accountable

One way that I like to hold myself accountable is by using the sleep metrics data on my Garmin fitness tracker. Fitness watches now do a decent job of monitoring your sleep patterns and allow you to monitor your data quickly and efficiently.

Most quality fitness trackers will track;

- The time you fell asleep
- The time you woke up
- The total time you slept
- The total time of "deep" sleep
- The total time of "light" sleep

This allows you to look at reports and statistics on your sleeping patterns. Are you going to bed at the same time each night? (Hello consistency!). Are you sleeping well? Are you getting your eight hours of sleep each night?

The fitness tracker is monitoring movement to approximate the sleep metrics. When you are awake, you are normally moving around (including your arms and your fitness tracker is attached to your wrist). If you are in a prolonged period of deep sleep, there is no movement. You are passed out. Your watch can assess your movements and make assumptions this way.

The point is, be honest with yourself. Use the data to get a better understanding of your sleep habits. If you aren't sleeping well, it makes obtaining health and wellness much more difficult.

So today, tomorrow, and then next day, say good-bye to the blue lights and implement these tricks into your daily routine. It's super Easy-Peasy this way. You can do it this way and it is sustainable.

It's all coming together. Keep up the good work. These little nuggets of knowledge and information are building up in your brain. Small 1% improvements are just stacking up on each other. You probably don't even realize how much progress you are making mentally, physically, and emotionally proceeding through this life transforming journey to optimum health because it is so Easy-Peasy.

Day 18 – Your Muscles Said, "Hey, Relax!"

Did you ever have one of those days where everything seems jacked up and stressful? Your boss is angry, your co-workers or customers are angry, your spouse is riding your butt and your kids are driving you bananas. The bills keep coming in the mail. The car breaks down unexpectedly. It appears you are running late for everything. When it rains, it pours, and the roof ends up leaking.

When these periods arise, your entire body tenses up. Your jaw starts to hurt. Maybe you even grind your teeth. Your neck starts getting sore and stiff. Your blood pressure rises. Headaches become a daily occurrence and you toss and turn all night trying to fall asleep.

Sometimes it appears life is a repeated set of kicks to the Tic-Tac's below the belt. Did you know that this type of tension can wreak havoc on your health and diet program? Wouldn't it be great if you could learn to relax more effectively?

But relaxing isn't as simple as it seems. And failure to relax can start a vicious circle where your health is impaired, and then you stress about your health being impaired, which causes even more stress.

Your ability to balance stress and relax will impact many other areas of your life. When you learn to control your stress better, you will be happier, have more energy, be more optimistic, maintain better relationships, think more clearly, and will be far more emotionally stable. You'll also be able to control your behaviors more and will be less likely to resort to consuming food, drink, or other bad things to help cope with the stress.

When you are stressed, your cortisol levels will rise (making weight loss far more difficult), you will age faster, run down your immune system, and be forced to deal with chronic inflammation.

Here are some tips on ways to calm down and relax every muscle in your body to reset your system;

1. If you have a decent sense of smell, aromatherapy has been proven to work. Research shows that scents of certain essential oils like lavender, chamomile, peppermint, and others can lower blood pressure and reduce anxiety. Spouses love flowers for more than the pretty looks. They make everything smell better.

2. Get a massage. This can be aided by a professional masseuse but trading massages with a significant other can work just as well. Massages can reduce pain, anxiety, and tension. It can also improve immunity defense. Even if you can sneak in and receive 10 or 15 minutes, every small bit can help improve the situation.

3. Do your 4-7-8 breathing exercises that were discussed on Day 11. 4 seconds of a deep inhale, hold it for 7 seconds, exhale for 8. Repeat that 4 times and if needed, do it multiple times a day.

4. Go for a walk. You need your steps anyway so lace up the shoes and get outside. Listen to some enjoyable music, a fun podcast, or just look around and be grateful for your blessings.

5. Take a hot bath with Epsom salts and/or essential oils. Hot baths have been used for thousands of years to aid in pain and relaxation.

6. Meditation and mindfulness. Learn to control your mind. Lay down on your back, take some deep breaths and think about every muscle just letting go and relaxing while the tension is eliminated.

Finally, use the power of "M" in your daily pursuit of stress management. Think about ways to simplify your life and make it less complex. Make small improvements on your finances, your health, your relationships, and your time management. Keep finding more ways to experience activities that bring joy and happiness to your life. That could be getting outdoors, reading a book, or enjoying time with friends.

Life is already hard, yet most people make it a lot harder than it should be because they are always finding new ways to complicate their lives. Instead, search and seek out ways to simplify. Less is more. Minimalism has an interesting way of delivering fulfillment.

So today, tomorrow, and the next day, work to simplify your life and get a better handle on your stress. Learn to stop and relax every muscle in your body from time to time. Incorporate this into your daily routine when it counts the most. It's super Easy-Peasy this way. You can do it this way and it is sustainable.

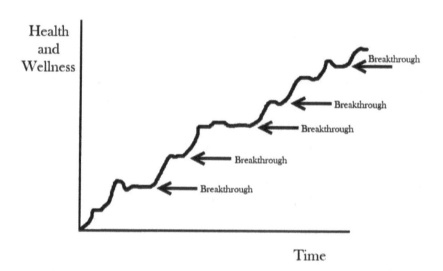

Day 19 – Believe That You Can Have Fun, Fun, Fun!

When I look back on previous seasons of my life, I now shake my head at what I was thinking and believing back then. I was brainwashed. I was misinformed. I was being manipulated.

You see, when I was in an unhealthy physical state, the kind where I had no energy, was overweight, and anxious about my future, I used food as a comforting and coping mechanism. I used to say things to myself like;

- "I deserve to eat this food (which meant ribs, soda, pizza, chocolate cake) because I had a hard day."
- "What fun is life if you can't enjoy good foods?"
- "I need to live a little. You only live once. I might as well enjoy my life."

The fact is, I had a lot of little sayings that I told myself to justify my eating and drinking choices. To make things worse and more difficult, I truly believed many of the things I was telling myself. I believed that if I didn't eat certain foods, I would be unhappy or even miserable in life. Who wants to live with that?

I believed that to have fun either by myself or with others, I needed to eat certain foods. I needed to eat chocolate cake. I needed to eat pizza until my head exploded (and my belly exploded).

And here's an interesting tidbit…When I tried to "quit eating bad foods," I couldn't do it. I'd only make it a few days or maybe a week or two and then I'd be right back to my old eating habits.

So, what changed? I did. I changed. SLOWLY. But even while changing slowly, I had to change certain things more dramatically. I had to get out of the mindset that I couldn't have a fun and happy life if I wasn't eating and drinking certain things. I had to change my beliefs that certain people wouldn't like me or would stop hanging out with me if I stopped eating certain foods like cake at every birthday party at work.

Now to be truthful, over time, some of my friends drifted off and I found new friends that shared the same new positive mindsets as I did. There were some people that wanted to stay stuck in the past which was unhealthy and unsustainable for me. That part of adapting to new healthier ways was scary.

When things are-a-changing, that means uncertainty. Uncertainty can easily transform into fear. It's the fear of the unknown that can play mind games with you. The reality is, humans like predictability even if it isn't a desirable situation.

That's why people stay in crappy jobs that they hate. Even though they hate their job and their boss, they know what to expect when they go into work every morning. So they stay, year after year. To leave would be to invite change into their lives and that leads to a lot of fear of the unknown.

That's the crazy part. Even though they hate their jobs now, they won't change because they fear hating their next job. But the only way to find a job that could bring more joy, satisfaction, and maybe even higher pay is to leave and change.

Fast forward a lot of years. I'm now a lot healthier, fit, and athletic than I was when I was in my 20's. I'm also a lot happier. I'm a lot more energetic. I'm a lot prouder of myself. Yet, I don't eat any of the crap that I consumed consistently when I was younger (and dumber). The reality is, the bad food that we eat is a false God. It doesn't lead to happiness. It leads to less happiness in the long-run. It's, "short-term satisfaction at the expense of long-term happiness."

That doesn't stop multinational and huge corporate conglomerates from spending billions of dollars trying to get us to eat their processed foods. Chips, alcohol, cakes, snacks, pizza's, frozen foods, and ice cream. The list is endless.

The more sugar and crap that we eat, the more revenue those companies earn. They are crafty enterprises. They make us feel that the food they sell us will make us happy. The ingredients that they add to processed foods are purposefully addictive. But the food they sell you doesn't make you healthy or happy over the long-term. They make you sick.

Which brings us back to a very important point on today's lesson and that is of personal beliefs. You must BELIEVE that you will be happier once you transform your health and wellness. You must BELIEVE that you will be more confident, more energetic, and more successful once you transform your health. You must BELIEVE that you are going to have MORE FUN, not less fun, once your body adapts to eating far more nutritious foods and drinks and you look and feel like a million dollars.

The secret is that the adaptive phase takes a bit of time. It's nothing you can't get through. It doesn't happen overnight. It didn't happen overnight for me and it won't happen overnight for you. But time will march on regardless, so you might as well end up where you desire.

Breaking a sugar addiction takes time and effort. Breaking an alcohol addiction takes time and effort. Breaking a sedentary lifestyle habit takes time and effort. Allowing your body to adapt to fruits, vegetables, nuts, seeds, and other sources of goodness doesn't happen overnight. But it is so worth it once you work through the process and come out the other side.

That is why so many people fail at this health situation. They don't make the transformation in a way that is **sustainable**. They don't slowly integrate new healthy foods **consistently**. They don't use the power of "**M**." They usually just try and switch their diet overnight in one big bang.

When their body freaks out, it experiences withdrawal symptoms. It's too much of a shock on the system. It's not used to all those new nutrients and it's not used to not getting the sugar, trans-fats, and chemicals that are in your processed foods that are so addictive.

The important point today is to BELIEVE in the bottom of your heart that you can have fun, fun, fun in life without all the crap in your diet. Imagine being a fit, energetic, and successful person that is living a good life. You will be able to do more things physically. Your brain will be sharper. Your energy will be higher. Your emotions will be more stable. You will be a ray of sunshine in the lives of others. You will have more fun once you complete this transformation.

And if you really want to think this through and convince yourself, imagine a fat and unhealthy person in your mind right now and ask yourself this, "How happy and how much fun are they really having in life?" Is that obese person really living the life of their dreams or are they just addicted to the foods that the big food corporations want them to purchase weekly at the grocery store? Are they happy buying expensive pills with all kinds of negative side effects that the pharmaceutical drug industry sells to help them cope?

So today, tomorrow, and the next day, have some fun, fun, fun without damaging your body and making yourself unhealthier. Visualize being a happy, confident, and proud person who loves eating clean and feeling magnificent. The energy that you will have will be unbelievable. Acknowledge that this transformation will take some time, but it is well worth the investment. It's super Easy-Peasy this way. You can do it this way and it is sustainable.

Daily Check-In

ARE YOU BUILDING MOMENTUM EACH DAY?

HOW DID YOU DO TODAY WITH YOUR GOALS?

- Did you reduce your sugar intake today?
- Did you eat some healthy foods?
- Did you get your daily steps?
- Did you get any sunshine and fresh air?
- Are you going to bed on time tonight?
- Did you take some steps to simplify your life?
- Did you crowd out something bad and substitute it for something good with your food?
- Did you reduce your exposure to bad influencers in your life?

Day 20 –Sugar and Other Hidden Addictions

Much of the developed world is slowly being overcome by addiction problems. Alcohol addictions, recreational drug addictions, and prescription drug addictions are some of the most widely known and discussed. But were you aware of the world's growing addiction to sugar? Yes, sugar. The supposedly harmless sweetener that is put in just about all processed foods and drinks and even cigarettes.

Consumption of sugar per person has skyrocketed over the last few decades. The average American consumes a whopping 66 pounds of sugar each year. It seems harmless enough. Who doesn't have a little sweet tooth? But did you know that research is now showing that sugar is an addictive intoxicant?

There are a few differences between addictions to other substances and addictions to sugar. First, the social stigma is different. Society has some sort of unwritten ranking scale as to the evilness of addictions. A crystal meth addiction is worse than a heroin addiction, which is worse than a cocaine addiction, which is worse than a pot addiction, which is worse than a tobacco addiction (which adds sugar to make them even more addictive), which is worse than an alcohol addiction (which also adds sugar to make the drinks more addictive), which is worse than a prescription drug addiction, which is worse than a sugar addiction. It's like a chain of addiction problems. Here's the deal, they are all harmful addictions with terrible long-term health benefits.

The second difference is that some addictions have more immediate short-term side effects. A crystal meth addiction doesn't take very long for a human being to become unwound with a myriad of physical, emotional, and behavioral problems.

Sugar on the other hand is more of a silent addiction with long-term side effects. You won't get pulled over for DUI from overloading on candy bars. You won't have slurred speech or be tempted to jump off tall buildings and believing you can fly while on a sugar high. But becoming addicted to eating candy bars and other common food sources with added sugar opens an entire host of health issues down the road.

Sugar induces many of the same responses in the region of the brain that acts as a reward center no different than nicotine, cocaine, heroin, and alcohol. Sugar stimulates the release of neurotransmitters, mainly dopamine. Sugar increases the physical craving for alcohol.

Many AA programs recommend the consumption of sweets and chocolate instead of alcohol when the cravings for alcohol arises. It's exchanging one addiction for another that may lead a person right back to the original addiction. Sugar just has a slower onslaught of long-term negative health consequences than the other.

Sugar is now put in almost all packaged and processed foods by those revenue hungry corporate conglomerates that want to sell you foods at a profit. Cookies, ice creams, sodas, cereals, salad dressings, sauces, soups, meats, and breads to name just a few. Do you think these companies are stupid? Do you think they are adding this sugar as a health benefit or as a profit building technique?

Sugar raises insulin and over time your body can develop insulin resistance. That is the primary driver of Type-2 diabetes, a condition that is now starting to impact children below 10 years of age. Sugar wreaks havoc on your physiological systems. Not only does insulin spike which causes negative hormonal changes that occur in chain reactions, but the empty calories just stack the deck in favor of prolonged and consistent weight gain over time. Bigger guts and bigger butts. Thank you sugar!

Once obesity sets in with diabetes, it's a death spiral. Obese and diabetic individuals have much higher risks of heart disease, cancer, strokes, and dementia. This is on top of becoming less and less healthy over time. How do you put a price tag on slowly losing your energy, your health, your confidence, and your self-esteem because of a growing gut and a growing butt?

Sugar is a slow, hidden, and undercover killer of our souls. You think it is making you happier in life. But it does the opposite. It's a dead-end. Sugar is the enemy.

Most people don't want to acknowledge sugar as the enemy. They try and justify it a million ways. They try and tell themselves that it is harmless and innocent, that it is ok to have a sweet tooth, that sugar leads to fun. They even reward their own children with it and often encourage them to consume it.

But those are false beliefs. It's the addiction talking. They may not even want to acknowledge that they have an addiction or treat their problem with the same severity of other harmful addictions. But the fact remains, sugar is the enemy.

Today is about becoming more aware of hidden addictions like sugar. There is a lot to learn and a lot to implement into your daily habits regarding sugar (and eliminating refined sugar from your diet). Like other areas of health, new habits must be formed.

You should make small changes to keep improvements sustainable. If something is sustainable, it could be done consistently. Anything that can be done consistently can lead to "M." "M" is the secret sauce. Anything is possible over time with "M."

So today, tomorrow, and the next day, start to become more aware of sugar in your diet. Read the list of ingredients in your processed foods. Begin to look for ways to crowd out highly processed foods with sugar for natural foods. The point isn't to eliminate fruit out of your diet. The point is to eliminate refined sugar out of your diet. Acknowledge that this transformation will take some time, but it is well worth the investment. It's super Easy-Peasy this way. You can do it this way and it is sustainable.

Health

Principles

ARE YOU BUILDING MOMENTUM EACH DAY?

THE FOUNDATIONS OF HEALTH SUCCESS

- Eat healthy
- Exercise your body
- Exercise your mind
- Exposure to sunshine and fresh air
- Get adequate sleep and rest
- Reduce stress and anxiety
- Avoid harmful substances (toxins, chemicals, drugs, alcohol, additives, and preservatives in foods.)

Day 21 –You Are Allowed To Smile During Exercise

As you know by now, I stress the importance of sustainability and consistency in taking on new habits and behaviors. It takes a certain amount of time for things to become second nature and automatic within our subconscious.

Once something becomes a habit, then that behavior becomes Easy-Peasy because there is no longer any resistance. Actions just happen as a part of our normal routine without any thought or extra effort. I like to joke and say that, "You'll start doing smart things repeatedly and you won't even know why."

Your brain wants to run what it considers its normal operating software. Your own operating software was developed based upon your daily routines that are unique to you and your life. Your operating software is different than your neighbors, or someone who lives in Africa, or practices a different religion in Hong Kong, or grew up in an Eskimo tribe in Alaska. Your brain created its own custom software based on your own unique life and what you exposed yourself to and decided to do.

Your brain doesn't want to work any harder than it must. Your brain is programmed to help you survive. It doesn't like getting clogged up with new code that requires extra energy and programming. That takes too much effort and energy.

Once you get things cooking in a good way and everything becomes automatic, then the magic really starts to happen. That's when the power of "M" really kicks in and the progress and transformation happens. **Momentum** is key. It's the secret sauce to success.

Many people discount or are completely ignorant of the power of "M." They also may ignore it in a rush for results. They want overnight success. They get impatient. They want immediate gratification. When I tell them that it doesn't matter how small they start on things, they often don't believe me. They want to fight that proven approach and start out much bigger and bolder.

This is so true when it comes to starting an exercise program that is meant to last a lifetime. I tell people to start with one push-up, one sit-up, or an easy walk down the street. I tell people to do a single squat or a walking lunge. They don't want to start small. They want to go big. They want to run 5 miles. They want to pump iron as if they were an accomplished bodybuilder.

They want to do a lot of exercise right away as if things were as easy as flipping on a light switch and turning on the energy. They expect that their brain will automatically and permanently run new operating software that hasn't even been written yet through repetition and consistency.

And look at where you are now. You are now on Day 21. It's the third week of the Easy-Peasy Health and Wellness approach. If you started small, your body would have already indicated to you that you could do just a tiny bit more "easily and sustainably" after the first week. Then a bit more after the second week. If you started with a single push-up, you are probably up to 3 pushups or 5 pushups. But it's **sustainable**.

You aren't doing anything that you can't do again the very next day. You don't want to overexert yourself where you must take a day off, stop your consistency and lose your momentum. It's too early for that.

Now compare yourself where you are now to the person who did it like everybody else and started out like gangbusters. After two weeks, most of them have already quit. They stopped, they flopped, and they failed.

They must start all over again which only becomes harder because of the psychological damage that was caused when they quit and failed at their previous attempt. They notched another mark in the failure column. How demoralizing is that?

How does that make them feel as they keep failing to make lasting change and they can't obtain the transformation that they seek? You are already ahead of everybody that took the gangbusters approach who quit already.

That should make you feel better about your progress because you have already passed by most people trying to make changes and we are only starting the third week of the program.

You put yourself on a path to success and they've already quit. Can you believe that???

Exercise Can Be Fun Too

I remind everybody that exercise doesn't have to feel like punishment. It doesn't have to be stripped of all fun. Exercise can be a lot of fun if you pick activities that you like. This may not be possible every single day but the more you can exercise and have fun, the easier it is to live a healthy lifestyle. You also knock out multiple life principles at once.

If you love playing tennis, play tennis. If you love playing golf, go golfing (just walk the course, don't take the cart). Fun exercise can be anything that keeps you moving and makes you use your muscles. Good exercise just needs to get your blood flowing and heart rate elevated, make you stretch a bit, move, and balance in unusual ways compared to your normal body routines.

I love doing martial arts and jiu-jitsu. It's just so much fun for me. I get to see my friends, practice the art, and have a lot of fun while getting in a fantastic workout. You don't have to do jiu-jitsu. Maybe you like hitting a heavy bag, lifting weights, dancing, kayaking, running, walking, golfing, tennis, kicking a ball around, or shooting hoops.

It doesn't matter what you like to do as much as it matters that you are having fun being active and making exercise an enjoyable endeavor. Playing physical games is fun and is exercise. Don't make this harder than it must be.

You may like doing things by yourself to enjoy quiet time where you can think or listen to a podcast. That's great. You may also like doing things with others where you get group social interaction.

I like mixing up a bit of both. There are times where I like walking on the treadmill by myself reading or listening to an audiobook. There are other times where I want to be with others and enjoy some competition and some laughs.

Whatever you choose, just be aware that you can smile during exercise. It's allowed. Exercise does not and should not be all about painful punishment. That's just not true. You can have fun doing physical activities that meet your needs. You just need to keep an open mind and search around a little bit for things that you may find interesting.

Don't be afraid of trying new things either. You may never know how much you will love something until you try that activity out. If you find an activity a little bit interesting or are curious about it, try it and see if you would like to do it more.

So today, tomorrow, and the next day, start to become more aware of how you can make exercise fun and enjoyable. Begin to look for ways to substitute boring things done by yourself with new fun things done with others. Have some laughs along the way.

BOOM! Easy-Peasy... Having fun and smiling during exercise leads to improved health and happiness. Who would have thought that you could gain so many health and wellness benefits from doing things that you enjoy and have fun at? You can see your friends, get in some social time, have some laughs, and get the blood pumping.

"A year from now you may wish you had started today." – *Karen Lamb*

Day 22 – YouTube'n Your Way To Health

Part of transforming yourself towards a life of health and wellness is acquiring new knowledge and information. It's all about learning new tricks, tidbits, techniques, and tactics. This new knowledge and information will allow you to discover what has worked for others so that you can learn to model that success and implement those processes into your own life.

Modeling allows you to learn quicker by observing others and seeing what works and how somebody else experienced breakthroughs for themselves. Modeling is a way to learn much quicker so that you don't have to go through or use the inefficient method of trial and error. Trial and error is far too inefficient and frustrating. It's also unnecessary. Others have already figured out how to live a life of health and wellness. There is no need to re-invent the wheel.

The easiest path to success is to find somebody else or a group of people that have already achieved whatever it is you want for yourself. The next step is to then breakdown and reverse engineer what it is they did or figured out in their own life so that you could implement that into your life. Modeling can save you years (or decades) because you can get right into the good stuff that made the difference in somebody else obtaining what it is that you want to obtain for yourself.

One of the best resources for doing this for health is to utilize the power of YouTube. YouTube has turned into a giant free life university where you can learn so many things for absolutely no charge. There is no tuition. There are no fees or expenses. You can go and search for just about anything and often find people that have not only learned how to do that particular thing, but are willing to give you tips and tricks for free.

This is certainly true in a lot of areas of health and wellness. You can learn so much on YouTube on items like cooking healthy, lifting weights, running, exercise, nutrition, motivation, weight loss, strength training, or doing all kinds of physical activities. It truly is amazing how much free information is on the internet from people that have reached their goals and figured out how to transform themselves.

Today is about taking the beginning steps to harness some of that information and knowledge that is on YouTube. Your task today is to get on YouTube and search out an area of health or wellness that is of interest to you. Search for anything that you are curious about.

Make this about you and not about what someone else is interested in. Listen to others, watch their examples, and learn from them. You will find all different kinds of styles, approaches, and personalities.

Use your spare time wisely and get in the habit of using YouTube as a resource for free knowledge and education on exercise tips, techniques, nutrition, cooking, learning more about vegetables, or different eating styles. The power of the internet is incredible. It's all right there at your fingertips and so much of it is also fun to watch and interesting to learn.

There are many people that are very generous with their time and are anxious to share their methods of success with you. They want you to improve your health and wellness.

Watching "how-to" videos on YouTube is one of the most entertaining and easy ways to increase knowledge, gather information, and stay motivated on your quest for personal improvement. The best part of it is that watching them is so EASY-PEASY!

So today, tomorrow, and the next day, start implementing some YouTube videos into your daily routine. It's super Easy-Peasy this way. You can do it this way and it is sustainable. Keep up the good work. You are changing and transforming yourself from the inside out.

Daily Check-In

ARE YOU BUILDING MOMENTUM EACH DAY?

HOW DID YOU DO TODAY WITH YOUR GOALS?

- Have you done any 4-7-8 breathing exercises today?
- Did you crowd out any bad foods and substitute them with "less bad" foods?
- Did you start the day with a healthy breakfast full of natural nutrients?
- Did you do just a tiny bit more exercise today than yesterday?
- Did you use your time wisely and listen to any podcasts or audiobooks while walking or driving in the car?
- Did you reduce your exposure to blue-lights an hour or two before bedtime?

Day 23 – Visualize The Future You

There is a paradox that I want to talk to you about today. It's a mental paradox. On one hand, the human brain is capable of amazing mental feats of intelligence, problem solving, and adaptability. Humans can problem solve, dream, and implement actions like no other creature on earth. The human brain can figure out how to build buildings, do math, invent cell phone technology, or how to fly a spacecraft to Mars. The human brain is remarkable.

But that same human brain is also capable of crippling itself with negative thoughts, polluted ideas, and enough stress and anxiety to cause actual physical harm to the rest of the physical body.

Stress and anxiety is the result of a brain that has become trained to be dependent on repeated thoughts of negative outlooks. Your brain is fully capable of making you miserable, making you feel inadequate, and making you feel like your future is hopeless. That darn annoying brain needs reprogramming to help you achieve whatever it is you want to achieve.

Fortunately, research confirms that your brain can be programmed to do all kinds of great things that enable you to live the good life that you deserve. Your brain is a lot like software. It runs repeatable programs that have been implemented by your habits. Your brain is likely to keep repeating the same thoughts that it held previously. This should be exciting news because research shows that you can substitute old thoughts with new thoughts and then get new results from those new thoughts! (That was a mouthful of a sentence).

Visualize

Research now shows that the secret key to achieving what you want in life lies in your ability to visualize it ahead of time. Top professional athletes have been using visualization techniques for years to enhance performance under pressure. Business professionals also use visualization techniques as they prepare for key speeches, presentations, and other important meetings.

The brain is wired to respond to mental imagery. The brain responds to those imaginary experiences like real world experiences. That's why athletes can experience the exact same physiological responses when they imagine that they are under a high-pressure situation with a game on the line. Their palms will get sweaty. Their blood pressure and heart rate will rise, and their breathing patterns will intensify.

The brain is responding to what the athlete is thinking about as if it is happening in real time. It starts to believe that the experience is real and responds accordingly with heightened awareness. The athlete will feel nervous as if thousands or millions of people are watching them perform.

You can learn to use this to your advantage. Your neural networks in your brain are being built and controlled by your thoughts. If you can think about success, imagine success, and visualize success, your brain will start building neural-networks to meet the needs required to achieve that success. In short, you start building substitute software for your brain to run that is built upon success principles rather than previously held bad habits.

The simple act of imagining success will help you achieve success. That's why top golfers will practice each shot in their mind before taking it, or basketball players will imagine making that free throw with the game on the line before taking it, or a musician will imagine playing the perfect song before performing it in front of a large concert audience.

This may sound all "woo-woo" but the research backs up this important point. What this means is that you must visualize health and wellness success as part of your health journey. You must imagine yourself being healthy. You must imagine what it will be like to eat healthy, be energized, and be fit. You must imagine what it will feel like to have the body that you want. You must visualize a whole new you before you can make that transformation in physical terms.

Mentally rehearsing success will help you stay on track and focused. Mentally rehearsing how you will respond when you are tired, stressed, and hungry can mean all the difference in the world when it requires you to make the right decisions for your own healthcare. You must envision eating the right foods every day. You must imagine exercising and feeling great about all that new energy you have. You must visualize what you will look like when you lose those pounds and need new clothes that fit you like a glove. You must visualize what it will feel like to look like a million dollars.

When you repeatedly imagine executing your processes and habits when performing health tasks, you are conditioning your neural pathways so that the actions feel familiar when you go to perform those tasks. You are training your brain to run on the new software.

Over time, those new thoughts and behaviors become the norm. They can be done without thought because you were performing tasks that were sustainable. That led to consistency which led to new habits. From there, everything led to improvement through the power of "M." Visualization can help ensure you are maximizing the power of "M" because you are imagining doing a little bit better every single day which leads you to doing a little bit better every single day.

Visualization can also greatly improve your stress and anxiety levels. Using meditation and visualization, imagine being more in control of your situation. Imagine and visualize being more calm, focused, and confident in your future. Visualize relaxing when problems arise as you know you can handle things with greater skill and energy.

So today, tomorrow and the next day, start implementing some new positive visualization techniques. Imagine what it will feel like when you are healthy. Imagine what it will feel like to have more energy. Imagine how proud you will be when you finally lose those excess pounds and keep them off permanently.

All it takes is a few moments of imagination to think of those images in your head. It's super Easy-Peasy this way. You can do it and it is sustainable. Keep up the good work. You are changing yourself from the inside-out.

Daily Check-In

ARE YOU BUILDING MOMENTUM EACH DAY?

HOW DID YOU DO TODAY WITH YOUR GOALS?

- Did you relax all of your muscles at least once today?
- Are you doing physical exercise that is more fun or enjoyable?
- Did you reduce your intake of processed sugar today?
- Did you watch any "how-to" videos on YouTube or other sources to learn how to model off of other successful health practitioners?
- Are you visualizing yourself as being a healthy and fit wellness practitioner?

Day 24 – The Good, The Bad, and The Ugly

Have you ever been at a social event where someone says to you, "Oh come on and have a drink, or a cookie, or a giant piece of cake? It's not going to kill you. You have to live a little and enjoy life, don't you?" It's like they are working overtime to try and get you to eat or drink something that is bad for you.

Have you ever stopped and wondered why people do this to each other? Why do most people encourage others to make the wrong choices instead of the right choices?

And why does it seem that all social events revolve around food and drinks that are more harmful to people than helpful?

That's why it is so important to be aware of who you are associating with daily. The reality is, you are often just like the five people that you are around the most. It's a lot easier for someone to bring a person down to their level than it is for someone to reach down and lift someone to a higher level.

Not all people are the same though. There are good influences, bad influences, and then just ugly influences. Each of these types of people should be dealt with differently.

Look, I'm not going to lie to you, people should surround themselves with as many good influences as possible. That goodness can and does rub off on others. Good people can provide words of encouragement, inspire you by being a good role model, or help you get back on track when you fall and need a pick-me-up.

Bad influences may not know any better. They may be just going with the flow or taking the path of least resistance. If everybody else is getting tanked or eating garbage food, they will just go with the flow and follow the crowd to fit in and be accepted.

Unfortunately, crowd pressures arise when the entire crowd is just going with the flow, but the flow isn't necessarily going in a positive direction. Then the entire group is having a negative impact on everybody associated with the group.

But then there is the last group of individuals which is the ugly. These are the people that intentionally go out of their way to slow you down, get in the way, or would gain satisfaction from watching you fail. These individuals are a magnet for trouble and offer you no positive benefits from being around them.

The thing about these negative, unproductive, unsuccessful people is that they are more than willing to throw out sharp tongued jabs, words of discouragement, or work extra overtime to get you to do something bad or harmful. But often it really isn't even about you at all. They are just trying to justify their own bad habits and bad behaviors because they don't know how to fix themselves.

Since they don't know or aren't willing to improve themselves, they would rather see others stuck in the mud pit with them. You know the saying, "Misery loves company."

How would it make these ugly souls feel if they encouraged you to do bad things to yourself, but you said, "No, I'm really working on improving myself and I am committed to positive change?" That puts them in a tough spot because they don't have the courage to change. If they see other people improving and working their way upwards on a success ladder, what is going to be their excuse then?

You need to pay attention for all three types of characters, the good, the bad, and the ugly. Surround yourself with as many positive influences as possible. It will make your path to success so much easier to be around like-minded individuals who are committed to personal excellence and health. They won't be discouraging you, they will be your biggest cheerleaders. They want you to succeed. They want you to reach your goals and follow your dreams.

The bad people need to be noted as well. If they are good people at heart but maybe don't know any better, there is a strong chance that they would love to improve themselves as well but just don't know how. You can lend them words of encouragement. You can be their cheerleader. You can help them reach their goals and help them climb up the ladder of success.

But if you note some of the ugly lost souls who are intentionally trying to hold you back, want to see you fail, or never have something good to say, these people need to be eliminated or put on the back burner in your life. They are nothing but trouble and need to be quarantined. You may not be able to eliminate them entirely, but you can be aware of what is going on and isolate yourself from their negative shenanigans as much as possible. Don't let them bring you down. That's what they want for themselves. That's not in your own self-interest.

Today is about taking an inventory of people in your life and trying to assess whether they are the good, the bad, or the ugly. Don't let others keep you from reaching your dreams and goals. Seek out others who are more than willing to help you succeed. They are there if you just keep an eye out for them. They certainly do exist in your community and on the internet.

There are plenty of people just like you who are interested in making a personal transformation and many people have already made that transformation happen and would love to share their journey with you.

So today, tomorrow, and the next day, start paying attention to those around you the most. Ask yourself if they are in the good, the bad, or the ugly buckets. Imagine how much better and easier your life would be if you were only surrounded by people that wanted you to succeed and wanted to help you reach your goals. Imagine how you would feel to know that you are surrounded by people that love you and will be so happy when you become fit and healthy.

All it takes is doing some inventory management and some understanding of who is in your life and how they impact you. It's super Easy-Peasy this way. You can do it and it is **sustainable**. Keep up the good work. You are changing yourself from the inside-out.

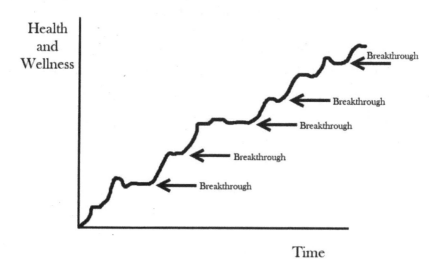

Day 25 – Eating Out Doesn't Have To Mean Pigging Out

Sometimes it's just nice to go out for a meal at a restaurant. This could be on weekends, special occasions, business lunches, or out of necessity when traveling. It's also nice for spouses who normally cook during the week to get a break and have somebody else wait on them, cook, and clean up.

Unfortunately for many, they take the wonderful opportunity to go out for a meal as an opportunity to make some bad choices for their health and wellness plans. Eating out to them means stuffing themselves to the gills. Some even eat a loaf of bread or a basket of tortilla chips before the meal is even served.

Once the meal is over, they barely have the capacity for any additional food in their stomach, so the desserts must be forced down with some intentional focus and hard work. This is when they seem to have the easiest ability to provide themselves with a positive affirmation like, "I CAN DO IT!" It's easy to eat far more than an entire day's worth of calories in a single session when dining out.

What do those who live healthy lives do for dining out meals? Do they not enjoy restaurants at all but rather stay home and eat cardboard with chia seeds sprinkled on top? Absolutely not. It's very possible to have a healthy lifestyle, eat clean, and stay fit even if you eat out at restaurants.

Here are some tips for when you want to dine out;

1. **Have a list of restaurants on hand ahead of time that can meet your nutritional and taste needs.** Let me give you an example. I eat lunch out every single day during the workweek. I eat gluten free and balanced nutritional meals are necessary. But I also like good tasting meals. If I need a nutritious lunch without breaking the bank or spending hours waiting for preparation and serving, I know I can hit up Panera Bread, Zoe's Kitchen, or Chipotle and have my needs met. I know I can make things work at Chick-Fil-A and multiple other restaurants as well. The point is, I know well ahead of time where I can (and do) go to get a good meal. I don't wait until the last minute when I'm starving to death, running late, or leave myself wondering, "Gosh, should I just stop at a pizzeria or some other fast food restaurant?" No way, no how!

2. **Have a list of menu items that are already on your personal "approved list."** We all have different preferences and tastes. Some like spicy foods, some like fish, some like chicken, and some like Mexican. It doesn't matter. What matters is that you know ahead of time not only what restaurants can meet your needs, but also what you will order once you get there. Don't wait until the server asks you, "Are you ready to order," to then cave in and get a greasy cheeseburger with fries and nachos because it sounded so good while you were starving to death waiting to order. Know what you want before arriving at the

restaurant. This prevents you from making bad decisions when the pressure is on. Write it down if you must. If you are going to a restaurant for the first time, look up the menu BEFORE you get there. Almost every restaurant has their full menu online along with nutritional specifications.

3. **Don't be afraid to ask for some help once you get there.** If you are in a jam at any decent restaurant, tell them what your specific eating goals are. If you are gluten free, allergic to shell fish, want a meat, a vegetable, a sweet potato, or salad, just tell them what you want. Most restaurants will do their best to accommodate customers. They want your business and very often customize per your desired specifications.

4. **Bring your own additions if necessary.** My wife and I call ourselves "hybrid diners." We enjoy going out to eat at restaurants, having full service, and not having to cook or clean up. We understand that not all restaurants can stock every item imaginable to our personal likings. Don't be afraid to take your own favorite healthy salad dressing or any other favorites in a little mason jar. Take nuts, seeds or organic berries for the top of your salad in place of croutons. Never be embarrassed about taking a few healthy items that can enhance your dining experience. Most restaurants want your business and want to see you enjoy yourself.

5. **Enjoy the dining out, the social interaction, and the service without feeling the need to damage your body.** After 15 minutes of you eating whatever it is you are going to eat, your body is going to register, "FULL." You have a choice

whether to fill the tanks with crap or nutritious items. Once you are full, your body is satisfied and wants to focus on digestion. Dining out is a wonderful convenience and experience that many people cannot do for budgetary reasons. Be grateful for having a great meal and not having to cook or clean. Enjoy your friends and family. For gosh sakes, have fun and enjoy the experience but walk away from the table without having to undue your pant buttons or loosen your belt.

6. **All you can eat does not mean eat all you can!** Next time you go to an all-u-can-eat buffet, look around at the other patrons and just ask yourself what their short or long-term health prognosis most likely is. It's terrible. Unless you are at an all-u-can-eat salad bar, avoid even putting yourself in situations where you are trying to please your wallet at the expense of your health. When diners go to an all-u-can-eat establishment, their mindset is to stuff themselves as much as possible to get the best value for their dollar. They obviously aren't factoring in their eventual healthcare costs to manage the upcoming heart disease, diabetes, and cancer by stuffing themselves with crap at the buffet. Don't be delusional. What you eat and how much you eat matters. The more you try and save money by eating at all-u-can-eat joints, the more you are going to have all kinds of crazy healthcare costs in the future repairing the long-term damage of your prior decisions. You aren't saving money. You are damaging your health and increasing your future healthcare costs.

7. **Who you eat out with sometimes matters.** We all influence each other. I'm lucky where my spouse is a nutritional expert and loves eating healthy. She is a positive influence on me because she sets an inspiring example of health and wellness. But not everybody is a source of inspiration, a role model, or a positive influence. Some people are the complete opposite. They have zero control over themselves. But not only are they terrible at managing themselves, they have that special knack to bring everybody around them down to their level. If they are drinking, they want everybody else to drink. If they are eating terrible, then everybody else goes down with the ship. Be careful who you associate with, socialize with, and dine out with. Your health may be dependent on it. And don't you believe for one minute that everybody out there is into personal gluttony whenever they dine out. That is not true. Plenty of people have learned how to dine out and eat nutritious meals. Dining out effectively is a learned skill and behavior.

Don't be afraid to dine out when necessary or if you want to dine out as a reward. Just use the opportunity wisely to monitor your finances and monitor your health requirements. You can do both while having a great time and enjoying the meals.

So today, tomorrow, and the next day, start implementing some good habits when dining out. Imagine what it will feel like to go out to eat with family and friends, have a ton of fun and enjoy a healthy meal. You will be so happy and proud of yourself when you come home that day. All it takes is just a little planning and focus to get prepared ahead of time.

It's super Easy-Peasy this way. You can do it and it is sustainable. Keep up the good work. You are changing yourself from the inside-out.

Day 26 – Find and Follow Mentors On The Internet

It's awesome when you could have people in your life that are wonderful positive influences and role models for you. These people can provide more than words of encouragement. They can provide you with all kinds of tips on what to do, when to do it, and how to do it. These are people that are a few (or many) levels above you on skills and experience in the health journey.

How did these people learn what and how to do things? The same way you will learn; reading, watching, talking to people, listening, experimenting, and observing. Some of it is trial and error but more importantly, it's learning how to implement proven processes of achievement into your life.

But what happens if you don't have any of these super-duper achievers in your day to day life? What happens if your friends and family are a step behind you and not willing to buck up and improve themselves right now or don't have the knowledge to help you? What happens if you feel all alone without having the ability to observe and learn from others live and in the flesh? What do you do then?

There's great news if this is the situation in your current life right now. There are LOTS of people on the internet that are just dying to show you how to make incremental improvements in your health journey. These people also have the goods to show for it. They are fit, healthy, energetic, motivating, and knowledgeable experts who know how to get results for themselves and for others. Sharing their knowledge is a passion of theirs and they do it through websites and other social media channels.

These experts regularly post blogs, produce how-to videos, use Twitter, Facebook, Instagram, and all kinds of digital tools to help share the goodness of their health and wellness message. There are many experts with various styles, personalities, and flavors that suit viewers of all different preferences. They share information that deals with all kinds of sub-sets of health and wellness such as;

- Nutrition
- Cooking and meal prep
- Time management
- Sport specific (running, triathlon, powerlifting, CrossFit, rowing, martial arts)
- Exercise specific (yoga, cardio, strength training, kettle bells, flexibility, mobility.)
- Mental focus, visualization, meditation
- Sleep and recovery

Some of these experts are old, young, men, women, funny, dry, technical, motivational, theoretical, philosophical. You name it, you can find it.

Now you might be saying, "But what's the point? Why do I need others?" Because having additional mentors who want to help you save time and succeed is a way to keep your learning Easy-Peasy. Why re-invent the wheel when others have already figured out how to do whatever it is you are struggling with right now.

More importantly, it's great to have inspirational and motivational messages available to you on a consistent basis. You will have plenty of highs and lows during your journey. Sometimes things will go smoothly while other times they will prove to be frustrating. Gains won't always come easy nor will gains always be linear. Sometimes you might even go backwards along your journey which will make you feel like quitting.

These mentors and thought leaders know what you are going through because they have experienced these rough patches and plateaus themselves. They know that sometimes it just takes a little extra push or extra words of encouragement or a new trick to get somebody unstuck and back on the path.

It's also fun to be part of a group of like-minded people and many of these mentors have other followers who are all going through the journey together. They may have private Facebook groups or forums or sponsor live webinars for you to participate in (ALL FOR FREE!)

The point is, the Internet is an outstanding resource for learning and motivation. Use the resources that are out there. Find some other people that are like your style, preferences, and personality. Not everybody wants to be a power-lifter or marathon runner. There is something for everybody. The key is to just keep making progress along your own health journey. Keep pushing yourself for those 1% improvements.

So today, tomorrow, and the next day, start searching around the internet for some role models and mentors that you find interesting who could help you learn even faster. Imagine what it will feel like to get those positive results with the confidence that you are doing practices that are proven winners. It's also a lot of fun as well as being super Easy-Peasy. You can do it and it is sustainable. Build that "M."

Keep up the good work. You are changing yourself from the inside-out. Be proud of yourself for taking the incremental steps of personal improvement.

Day 27 – What To Avoid When You Want Some Awesome Snoozers

You continue to make awesome progress on your 30 Days To Health and Wellness the Easy-Peasy Way. You know that sleep and recovery is one of the key principles of health and wellness. Sleep and recovery impacts your health, your energy levels, your potential during workouts, your emotions, and your overall happiness.

Without adequate sleep, living a life of health and wellness is simply impossible. Yet, so many people ignore this principle of health or are uninformed on ways to make improvements in this area.

You already learned on Day 17 about blue-light coming from electronics like TV's, smartphones, tablet computers, and laptops. Those are to be avoided a few hours before going to bed (unless you wear blue light blocking glasses).

There are also other helpful practices that can impact the quality of your sleep which include;

- Regular sleeping hours which require you to go to bed and wake up at the same approximate time each day.

- Darken the room. Quality of sleep can improve if you eliminate light that may be telling your body that it is time to be awake.
- Temperature of the room. Cooler room temperature has been shown to increase the quality of sleep. Look to set your room temperature between 60 and 68 degrees.
- Noise. Cut out all the unnecessary noise that you have control over. That may not be possible if you live near an airport or train station or live in a busy city but be aware that noisy environments that impact your sleep will eventually impact your life. Choose wisely on how you want to live your life. Big city living that runs 24/7 may be a hoot right up until you experience cardiac arrest at 45 years old.
- Quality mattress. There is no better investment than a quality mattress. Think about it, if your goal is to sleep 8 hours a day and we have 24 hours in a day, that means 1/3 of each day is spent in bed. That equates to 1/3 of your life. Why wouldn't you spend the time and money required to figure out the perfect mattress? What other item in your life will you use this much? How much money do you spend/waste on items that are used far less? Choose wisely. Invest in a quality bed, mattress, pillows, and sheets.

Beyond these items, here is a short list of items to monitor as you work towards boosting the amount of quality and quantity of sleep;

1. **Prescription Medications**. Hopefully you aren't in need of these. If you are, that's a sign that your body and health are already starting to fail you in unnatural ways. But if you are using prescription medications, note that many medicines and nutritional supplements can impact the amount and quality of sleep you get. Ask your doctor about plans to reduce and eliminate the need for prescription medications if possible.

2. **Caffeine**. Caffeine can show up in all kinds of places. It usually shows up in beverages like coffee, tea, sodas, and energy drinks (all the things people drink because they need more energy due to lack of sleep). But caffeine can also show up in foods like chocolate, ice cream, energy bars, yogurt, and even "decaffeinated coffee." Caffeine can stay in the system for more than 12 hours. That means lunchtime drinks can impact your sleep.

3. **Chocolate**. Chocolate may not only include caffeine, but many high-quality dark chocolates (including the healthy kinds) contain the stimulant theobromine which increases heart rate and impacts sleep. Theobromine can stay in the system for longer than 18 hours which means even chocolate at lunch or in the morning can impact your sleep that night.

4. **Spicy and fatty foods**. Spicy foods can impact acid reflux and that isn't going to help you get quality sleep when the lights go out.

5. **Alcohol**. The interesting thing about alcohol is that many people believe it can help them sleep because alcohol can make them feel drowsy. But sleep is reduced when the body is working on metabolizing the alcohol. Alcohol has been shown to help people fall asleep faster, but it reduces REM and the quality of your sleep. Don't booze it up before bedtime. (Don't booze it up at all if you know what is good for you).

6. **Sugar**. Getting jacked up on sugar isn't going to help you sleep. It's going to give you a sugar high and keep you buzzing for hours. You wouldn't give a kid candy before going to bed so put down the Twizzlers and cupcakes and skip the empty calories before bedtime.

7. **Recreational drugs**. Uhhh duh. You would think this would be obvious but "Just say no." There's a difference between getting quality sleep and passing out from escape drugs.

8. **Stress**. Are you worried and anxious? There are methods to quiet the mind before bedtime to improve your odds of improving the quality and quantity of sleep. Meditate prior to bedtime with the help of free meditation apps on your smartphone. Use lavender or other essential oils on your sheets and pillow cases. Take a warm bath before bedtime to calm yourself. Listen to peaceful music while using mental imagery of enjoyable surroundings like the beach, mountains, or desirable places.

You would think that sleeping would be easy for many people (it sure seems easy for college kids in their classes). But the fact is, as we age, many people find it harder and harder to experience getting quality sleep in adequate quantities. That's why it pays to monitor all the details that go into getting quality sleep. Your health depends on it.

So today, tomorrow, and the next day, start paying attention to items that you may be consuming during the afternoon and evening hours that are known to impact the quality of your sleep. Imagine what it will feel like to get a super night's sleep where you wake up energized and ready to attack the next day. Imagine feeling great during your workouts, and household chores, and at work.

Sleeping should be an easy item to accomplish (all you must do is just lay there, it's not like lifting weights or running a marathon.)

Keep up the good work. You are changing yourself from the inside-out. Be proud of all your progress and incremental gains. You are on your way to personal achievement and reaching your goals.

Daily Check-In

ARE YOU BUILDING MOMENTUM EACH DAY?

HOW DID YOU DO TODAY WITH YOUR GOALS?

- Are you surrounding yourself with people that are positive influencers and reducing time with those that are negative influencers?
- Did you pre-plan your dining and eating strategies to make sure you don't sabotage your health goals?
- Did you seek out and follow any mentors including the internet that could act as role models for success?
- Did you avoid the major impediments to getting quality sleep today?

Day 28 – Simplifying Your Life To The Basic Essentials Of Success

Life is hard. Sometimes it's really hard. That's just all part of the human experience. We all must navigate speed bumps, obstacles, setbacks, and outright failures. These life episodes set us back, cost us time, drain us of our energy and sap our confidence.

John Wayne (The Duke) use to joke, "Life is hard. It's even harder if you're stupid."

I often say, "Life is hard. It's even harder when you work overtime to make your life far more complicated than it has to be."

Life in the developed world has a knack for sucking us into increasingly complicated situations. Without personal reflection and correction, we wake up to realize that we are not following proven principles of success. As we learned, principles of success aren't complicated items or hard to understand. Most principles are quite simple to understand. The difficulty is setting up your life in a way that you can follow simple principles.

As most people will attest, they find difficulty in this task as their lives get increasingly complicated. Usually, they are not living by any of the proven principles of success. They aren't using principles as a guide to help them make the best decisions for their own long-term self-interest. Principles should act as your compass, giving you guidance on what the best decision is based on your desired outcomes in life.

As a review, we learned that the principles of success in health and wellness are as follows;

1. Eat healthy
2. Exercise your body
3. Exercise your mind
4. Exposure to sunshine and fresh air
5. Get adequate sleep and rest
6. Reduce stress and anxiety
7. Avoid harmful substances (toxins, chemicals, drugs, alcohol, additives, and preservatives in foods.)

As you can see, none of those concepts are difficult to understand. But how often are you proceeding through your days using these principles to guide you? Have you ever stopped and reflected on how complicated your life has become and why?

Complicated lives happen in a lot of situations. Here are a few examples;

- Someone spends more money than they make. To float the deficits, they take on a little debt, then a little more,

then a little more. Soon, the debt overwhelms them, and
they become trapped. Then they are forced to keep
working jobs that they hate to keep their heads above
water which only keeps getting more difficult over time.
Life becomes complicated.

- Someone has complicated relationships and find
  themselves always fighting and being in combative
  situations with others. Their social circles are filled with
  people that act as bad influences on one another. They
  spend a lot of excess time on managing poor
  relationships rather than on fun or productive activities.
  It becomes exhausting (and complicated).
- Someone ignores their health until alas, their health
  starts to ignore them. Life quickly becomes complicated.
- Someone over-commits to too many things and spreads
  themselves too thin. It ends up making them feel that
  they are always behind, running late, and can't find the
  time to squeeze everything in. Life becomes
  complicated.
- Rather than finding a few activities that add authentic
  joy to their lives, they chase activities that add up to
  being complicated, expensive, and hard to pull off
  logistically on a consistent basis. Life becomes
  complicated.

The research on happiness ends up being counter-intuitive.
Those that often live in the wealthiest nations and communities,
often end up being less happy than others with less material

and luxury items. That seems to be the trend in America for sure. American's on average are wealthier than all other nations, yet, we are the most over-worked, stressed, and anxious. We are certainly not the happiest culture.

How is it that with each passing year as adults, we add, "just a bit more complication to our lives?" The increase is small, but steady. Day by day, week by week, year by year. Like a dripping faucet, drip, drip, drip. Each drip is one more commitment, on more monthly bill, or one more purchased good that needs maintenance. One day we wake up to one heck of a complicated life. "How did this happen?" we ask ourselves.

The reality is, these complications add up to a lot of burdens, a lot of headaches, and a lot of time commitments. These complications lead to stress and anxiety. Stress and anxiety often leads to making bad food and drink choices. We start looking for escapes in all the wrong places like cigarettes, alcohol, or worse – drugs.

Being over-committed to things means we are not in control of our time. That means no to workouts and exercise. That means little time for reading, listening to music, or watching things that lead to increased knowledge and information regarding our health. That means little time to find new friends and expand our social circles. That means trying to buy our happiness with impulsive purchases on material items that lose their luster after a short time. Then we move on to our next purchase to chase happiness. Money starts slipping out of our pockets.

What we often see is an inverse relationship between a healthy life and a complicated life. The more complicated we make things, the more our health seems to slip away. What can you do to reverse this? You must simplify!

The more things you can eliminate, the more you can detach from, the more you can simplify, the easier it will be to live a healthy (and happy) life. Work to reduce your bills. Work to get rid of unused items. Work to free up your schedule. Work to find friends who are positive role models in your life.

So today, tomorrow, and then next day, start paying attention to areas of your life that are complicated that need attention. Work little by little to simplify your life. Work to free up time. Work to reduce your expenses. Work to create and maintain excellent relationships with people. Simplifying your life will allow you to live a life of health and wellness.

Keep up the good work. You are changing yourself from the inside-out little by little. These changes keep adding up. You are being consistent and building momentum. Be proud of the incremental progress and gains. You are well on your way to personal achievement and reaching your goals. You are on your way to the health that you deserve and desire.

Health

Principles

ARE YOU BUILDING MOMENTUM EACH DAY?

THE FOUNDATIONS OF HEALTH SUCCESS

- Eat healthy
- Exercise your body
- Exercise your mind
- Exposure to sunshine and fresh air
- Get adequate sleep and rest
- Reduce stress and anxiety
- Avoid harmful substances (toxins, chemicals, drugs, alcohol, additives, and preservatives in foods.)

Day 29 – Hairpin Triggers

Are you aware of what your "hairpin triggers" are? If you were a gun lover, your definition of a hairpin trigger would be more of a hair trigger. It's a modification made to a gun which makes it respond to very little pressure on the trigger. The slightest pull of the finger, and "BOOM!" the gun fires.

In life, there are situations that can greatly impact our emotions. These are emotional hairpin triggers. These are feelings we get that can be destabilizing to our emotional well-being. These emotional hairpin triggers can often be initiated by several sources resulting in an emotional "BOOM" that often lead to negative health consequences. Some examples might include;

- Certain statements that your boss or co-workers say to you.
- The way a family member treats you.
- Money issues.
- Traffic.
- Scheduling and time conflicts.
- Guilt or feeling inadequate about yourself or your life.
- Experiencing failure.

When our hairpin emotional triggers are initiated, it can start an entire process or chain reaction with negative consequences. We can experience higher blood pressure, anger, fear, depression, lose sleep, feel shame, or withdraw from social circles. Being in such a negative state can also lead to making bad decisions.

Triggers can increase our desire to avoid painful feelings by suppressing them with items like bad foods (candy, ice-cream, cookies, cakes, or other junk food), alcohol, drugs, or staying in bed. When these painful feelings are triggered, it's much more likely that your behaviors or habits are going to impact the progress you are making on your health and wellness journey.

It's not unusual for triggers to not only halt all progress and momentum on our health journey, but they may turn us around where we start going backwards. Going backwards is deflating, defeating, and makes us feel like we are never going to reach our health goals. We can dig ourselves a hole and make matters much worse than they should be. That makes it much more likely to continue with follow-up bad behaviors and actions. Things can quickly escalate into a downward spiral.

The quicker you can identify and connect your triggers, the more effective you can be at doing preemptive strikes against them to ensure that you nip things in the butt before things spiral out of control. You can learn how to recognize the trigger and then direct energy towards managing positive outcomes and avoiding negative behaviors that will only sabotage your success principles.

We all have triggers that can lead to impatience, anger, and frustration. How we deal with these triggers is essential for us to navigate our lives in a way that allows us to pursue the health and wellness that we desire and deserve.

Ultimately, we are striving for lower blood pressure, lower blood sugar, healthy diets, high energy, good exercise, quality sleep, and peace in our lives. The next time you have a set-back, ask yourself with reflection why the set-back occurred. What triggered the negative response? Make a mental note of the series of events that led to the trigger so you can step in and avoid making the same decisions the next time it occurs.

So today, tomorrow, and the next day, start paying attention to the specific times where you experienced a hairpin trigger that led to poor health decisions. Imagine different options that you could have done to make yourself feel differently about your long-term goals and objectives.

You never want to put yourself in positions where you dig yourself into a deeper hole. We all have set-backs. We all experience failures. How we respond to those set-backs and failures makes all the difference in the world.

"When you find yourself in a hole, the first step in getting out is to stop digging deeper. Just put the shovel down."

Keep up the good work. You are continuing to make progress with each passing day. With consistency, these incremental improvements add up to life changing results. Be proud of yourself for acting, focusing on personal change, and moving towards personal improvement.

Build Momentum

Breakthroughs

Track Results

Start Now

Eat Healthy Foods

Sunshine and Fresh Air

Take A Deep Breath

Create Processes

CROWD OUT AND SUBSTITUTE

EXERCISE DAILY

PROVEN PRINCIPLES

Just A Tiny Bit More Than Yesterday

Develop Better Habits

Avoid Sleep Destroyers

Simplify Your Life

Morning Rocket Fuel

Learn Your Hairpin Triggers

Learn From YouTube

FOLLOW MENTORS

Visualize The Future You

Eat Out Wisely

Reduce The Sugar

Have Fun While Exercising

NO BLUE LIGHTS BEFORE BED

Relax The Muscles

ADEQUATE SLEEP

Listen To A Good Podcast

Day 30 – Holy Schnikees! You Did It! Now What?

Congratulations! You did it! You completed the 30 Days To Better Health The Easy-Peasy Way. This is just one step of many along your path to health and wellness.

Completing the 30 days often comes with mixed emotions. It's a mix of excitement for having completed something along with a bit of the wind exiting the sails. You may feel as though the end is anti-climactic. It's 30 days later, yet it dawns on you;

- You still aren't Superman or Wonder Woman.
- You didn't lose 60 pounds in 30 days.
- You didn't resolve all your health items that need attention.
- Maybe some other people in your life didn't even notice one physical change in you (yet).
- You don't even understand how much knowledge and information you learned that will set yourself up for permanent success.

But guess what? That's all part of the process. That is all 100% normal and expected. It is important to realize that there is no perfection. There is only "better" or "worse." You want to do more of "better" and less of "worse."

Time will pass by no matter what you choose to do. 30 days have already passed. Another 30 days will be behind you soon enough. And another 30 days after that. That's why you need to use the time that you do have as effectively and efficiently as possible.

Let's talk about all the wonderful things that did happen. First off, isn't it amazing how fast 30 days can go by? It seems like you were just working on the first few days of the cycle, getting set up, talking about measurements and metrics. Second, if you made it this far (and you did since you are reading this chapter), you have already made it longer than all those people that start out on a new program guns-a-blazing only to flame out and quit after a week or two.

But not you. You used perseverance and outlasted all the quitters who tried yet again to do something that didn't work. They bit off more than they could chew, they tried to do everything at once, and then they folded like a cheap tent on a camping trip. They never built into their program **momentum** based on what can be done **consistently** and **sustainably**. They never changed their long-term **habits**.

The fact is, if you did all the daily readings and even implemented a fraction of the knowledge and information, you blew away the competition. Let's get into what you now know that they still don't. Trust me, you are going to be impressed with yourself once you see how all of this came together. You are WAYYYY ahead of the curve and you probably didn't even grasp the importance of it.

What's Your Why?

During this process, you gained a better understanding of yourself and "why" improving your health is so important to you. "Why" now? "Why" change? "Why" lose weight? "Why" are you more motivated than ever to finally get lasting changes that you deserve? The more clarity you have on your own "why", the more you can stay focused on staying the course, work through obstacles, and achieve the personal success that you deserve.

Knowledge and Information – The "What"

During this journey of Easy-Peasy health, you obtained a lot of essential knowledge and information that is the foundation of "what" to do. This knowledge and information is critical as it guides you on doing more of what we know works and doing less of what doesn't work.   Part of this process is acknowledging that what you were doing in the past is in fact not providing you the results that you seek deep down.

Acknowledging your past is important to come to grips with because if you kept doing the same things you did in the past, you would keep getting the same old results. But you don't want those old results. You want new improved results. You want change. You want personal transformation that will last a lifetime. New results require doing new things. That's why the knowledge and information is important, so you learn "what" to do and "what" not to do.

Proven Principles

The knowledge and information provided to you that will help you get your intended results is based on proven principles of health and wellness. These principles are timeless and your ability to implement the principles will mean the difference between success and failure. The most important principles for your health and wellness that we covered along with specific sub-topics are;

1. Eating healthy – what to eat, what not to eat
   a. You were provided a chart in Day 6 of what to eat and what not to eat to get you started moving in the right direction.
   b. The importance of starting the day with a proper morning breakfast and how to slowly transition towards a high-powered breakfast.
   c. How sugar can be just as addictive as alcohol and drugs.
   d. Eating out doesn't mean pigging out.
2. Exercise the body
   a. Starting small and using the power of "M" to achieve awesome results that last a lifetime.
   b. How to concentrate on developing habits first, then increase workload second.
   c. How exercise can be fun and social.
3. Exercise the mind

    a. The importance of reading books and articles on health and wellness.

    b. Listening to podcasts to kill two birds with one stone.

    c. Watching YouTube videos to learn new tricks and techniques.

    d. How following others on social media can inspire you and provide you with additional role models of success.

4. The importance of sunshine and fresh air on our health and wellness.

    a. Get some free energy.

    b. Get a natural dose of Vitamin D.

    c. Reduce stress and depression.

    d. Enjoy physical activities with friends and family.

5. Adequate sleep, rest, and recovery

    a. Setting regular sleeping hours and striving for at least 8 hours per night of quality sleep.

    b. How blue light from electronics can disrupt your circadian rhythm.

    c. Using technology as a tool to track your sleep for an honest assessment of your situation.

    d. Avoiding certain foods, caffeine, drugs, alcohol, and sugar well prior to going to bed.

6. Reducing stress

    a. How 4-7-8 breathing can help reset your mental state and reduce stress and anxiety overload.

    b. Periodically relaxing every muscle in your body.

    c. Meditating and visualizing success.

    d. The importance of simplifying your life and reducing complications.
7. Avoiding harmful substances
    a. How to "crowd out" and use the technique of "substitution."
    b. You can have fun in life without damaging yourself.
    c. Avoiding and reducing exposure to bad influencers.
    d. Learn to identify and manage your emotional triggers

You now know that the 30-day Easy-Peasy process deals with implementing the principles of success. Mastery of the principles will take time and many rounds of the 30-day process. But the good news is that you are now working a program that leads to lasting and permanent success. This isn't about a fad diet or short-term trend. This is a success program that is about building a lasting lifestyle in winning the health battle that will reward you until your end of days.

As you work towards implementing all the success principles, you are taking an approach that will work over the long-term. That means you aren't trying to turn your entire life upside down and shock your system in any way that is unsustainable.

You'll also have more peace and patience with yourself because you aren't working around fabricated or unrealistic expectations about getting results in 10 days or some crazy gimmick. It took you a long time to get to this point in your life. Fortunately, it takes far less time to get positive results than it did to get you to where you are now.

Sustainable and Consistent Actions

Everything that you are working on now and in the future must be **sustainable**. If you are making small improvements that are sustainable, you will be able to implement those changes **consistently**.   Anything that is done consistently will eventually turn into **habit**. Habits are powerful because once something is a habit, you can do it automatically with zero thought or effort. It becomes mindless and without resistance.

A Habit of Success

Habits work both ways because you can implement good habits or bad habits. What you do for most of your waking hours is done on auto-pilot through habits. You wake up and start doing the exact same things repeatedly without even thinking about them. Replacing bad habits with good habits is essential for success in any endeavor. During each 30-day cycle, you are making small incremental changes that lead to new and improved habits. These new habits just keep stacking up one on top of the other and snowball into a mountain of success.

Adaptive Bodies and Minds

Implementing good habits is possible because the human body is **adaptive**. The human body adjusts and adapts to most things that it is exposed to **repetitively**. That's why Eskimo's can live in cold climates, drug addicts can keep doing drugs, or why somebody else needs to run 10 miles a day. The body adapts to what it learns to do through habit. Your goal is to make your body adapt to positive changes and away from negative influences and behaviors.

The Power of "M"

By doing things that are **sustainable** you will build **consistency**. Consistency leads to **habits**. Consistency allows you to make small never-ending improvements that build "**M**." "M" is the secret sauce. **Momentum** is the magic that makes everything happen because with "M" anything is possible. Small 1% improvements add up to huge changes over time. Every breakthrough in human performance happens through "M." "M" can't happen without good habits that lead to consistency.   You are looking to achieve small 1% improvements each day that just keep stacking up one on top of the other.

You Have To Believe It To Achieve It

Success requires the support of an internal belief system. You must believe you can change. You must visualize yourself living a happy life as a healthy person. You may not know exactly how good it feels to be healthy, fit, and energetic right now, but you must have faith that it is SOOO much better than being unhealthy, lethargic, and on track for all kinds of chronic diseases.

Every 60 seconds someone in the United States develops a chronic disease. Per the Center For Disease Control (CDC), chronic diseases are responsible for 7 out of every 10 deaths. Don't let it be you. Most of these are avoidable diseases. You can be successful. You must believe it to achieve it.

The 30-Days To Better Health The Easy-Peasy Way focuses on the "what" portion of health and wellness. It is acquiring the core knowledge and understanding of how you are building a new life supported by proven principles of health and fitness. That foundation will allow you to build upwards from there. It's no different than building a big and strong pyramid. You can't build up and live a life of your dreams without a strong base and foundation.

What To Do Now?

That's an easy question to answer. The thing to do now is start over again with the 30-day cycle. Go back to the beginning. It's time to take measurements and gather your updated metrics. It's time to go through everything again but this time, you will have the opportunity to get something new out of the exact same information. You will have another opportunity to make small improvements in every category along the way. There is no perfection, only a process and progress towards mastery.

The principles are always the same. But our life is constantly changing, and we are always seeking to gain new knowledge and information that can be applied towards implementing the proven principles of success in health and wellness.

This is also a good time to ask any questions that you have. What are you stuck on? What didn't make sense? What were the most difficult things to implement in this 30-day cycle? Let me know how you are doing and how the small changes are starting to add up. You can contact me through my website at www.paulkindzia.com

As you know, one way or another, 30-days is going to pass by. Where will you be after another cycle? The other good thing is that when you have setbacks, know that you can work on making improvements in that area in the very next 30-day cycle.

Congratulations again on making progress on your journey. You should celebrate and acknowledge yourself and your efforts (just not with harmful food, drinks, and substances. You learned why to avoid those now). It's all coming together for you bit by bit.

Bonus Chapter 1 - The Haters, Baiters, And Non-Believers

Unfortunately, health and wellness aren't always an easy task to achieve within your own family and social circles. That may sound odd, but it is true. The fact is, not everybody will want you to succeed, but it will be for various reasons that may not have occurred to you before starting your journey. You will experience many social circumstances along the way, so it's best to be prepared for those ahead of time.

Being aware of health-related social circumstances will allow you the opportunities to stay focused and to have the confidence that you are indeed doing the right tactics FOR YOU.

Listed below are three types of individuals with whom you will cross paths with along your journey. It will benefit you to understand these personality behaviors ahead of your encounters with them. Knowledge of their typical behaviors will allow you to navigate social situations in pursuit of your health goals with greater ease and comfort.

Haters Are Going To Hate

"Everybody loves a good success story, unless it's not their own."
– Paul Kindzia

Haters tend to want to knock another person down a few notches. This vitriol or bitterness could come in many different forms, such as a snotty comment, a glance of disdain with rolling of the eyes, or gossip among your peer group. Haters are like the trolls on the internet who would rather spend their limited time on earth bringing somebody else down or criticizing another person rather than spending that time to improve their personal situation.

Humans have a behavioral tendency to believe that each of us is at the center of our own universe. Further, it's human tendency to compare our universe against the universes of those closest to us in social or family relationships. It's in our nature to compete. Competition is nature's way of working her magic where the strong survive and pass on the best genetics.

Instinct makes us compete. We compete for food and jobs. We compete for material possessions. But at our core, we compete for sex, mates, and social status. It just so happens that humans have evolved in ways that aren't as obvious as peacock feathers and elk antlers to display superiority among competitors. Rather than long and colorful peacock feathers to display our excellence, humans implement a mix of material possessions such as clothes, cars, jewelry, or houses to display their social ranking along with perceived health (hence the huge plastic surgery industry – why achieve real health when you can slice and dice and use liposuction and other expensive and dangerous surgeries?)

At its core, money and the appearance of health represents success and power for men along with power and security for women. It's in our DNA. Men want to be strong, powerful, and successful. Doing so increases their odds in attracting those of the opposite sex (Men, how often have we seen TV infomercials selling us a bulging muscles and six-pack abs schemes so, "You too can have a bikini-clad bombshell on your arms!")

Women are attracted to strong, powerful, successful men as it provides the best chances of security that is programmed into their DNA. The purpose of stating this (which may appear to be obvious by some) isn't to create a social argument. Women and men alike can be very healthy and happy. Women can be strong, powerful, and successful. The point is to understand human behavior at its core.

When you move up the health ladder, you are altering the current dynamics of your social circles and peer groups. If you move up, well then what does that mean for those who now are below you on a health scale? What are they going to think of the situation? Are they going to go out of their way to say, "Congratulations for making me look less attractive to my peers, co-workers, company leaders, family members, community, and my potential mates?"

You will have a trim midsection, they will have a muffin-top or beer belly.

Haters won't be able to match your real output or progress. Therefore, they are limited by words or actions against you. The best thing you can do is accept it as a sign of achievement. Remember, you aren't trying to make others look bad. You are trying to improve yourself and make progress along your journey.

There will be breakthroughs that you achieve along the way that will be noticed by others during your journey. This is certainly the case when getting in shape and working out. After two days of working out, others aren't going to notice anything different about you. But after a few weeks, they will begin to say, "There is something different about him/her." After a few months, it's clear to everybody, "That person has it going on!"

When you get in better physical shape, it's more than just visual. It changes your soul. You know you evolved into a different person, and thus, you carry yourself differently. You will become more confident. You will become more content. You will become more energetic. You will feel the changes and others will notice it as well.

I want to share one tidbit that relates to haters. This tidbit comes from Coach Nick Saban, one of the winningest college football coaches of all time. He has coached national championship teams at different universities and was rated by Forbes Magazine in 2008 as "The Most Powerful Coach in Sports." Here's what Nick Saban would share with his teams:

"Mediocre people don't like high achievers. High achievers don't like mediocre people." – Nick Saban

You always see interesting human social dynamics when you start mixing high achievers with low achievers. Both will be annoyed with the other side but for the opposite reasons. You need to decide which camp you want to settle in and go from there.

When haters hate, be patient, be proud, and understand the deeper context of the situation to avoid conflict.

Baiters

Baiters create a different social dynamic than haters. A Baiter is somebody within your family, peer group, or social circle who tries to entice you to make bad health decisions.

Have you ever been on a diet and the people around you constantly make comments like, "Just have one, "or "You can have a little," or "But it's a birthday party, so eat some cake. Life is short, so enjoy!"

Those are Baiters.

Staying true to your health plan is hard. But when you see your family, friends, neighbors, and co-workers eating, drinking, and doing other bad things like it is New Year's Eve, it may become tremendously hard to execute your health and wellness plans. Your feelings, determination, and focus can deteriorate when people whom you either like or are forced to be around due to social dynamics place pressure on you – either subtle or not-so-subtle – to throw your health plans out the window and "eat the proverbial chocolate cake for breakfast."

It is essential that you visualize and rehearse for these social situations, which are bound to arise and can make you feel quite awkward. What do you do when everybody at work says, "We are going out for dinner and drinks after work. Do you want to come?" and you say, "I'm not indulging in the extra calories. I have a weight loss goal this month."

What does this imply to the others?

It's important that you are sensitive to others with whom you spend time along your journey. Most people struggle with health and weight issues. People think about their physical appearance and how they feel more than almost any other issue in their lives. When you say, "Hey, I've got goals; I've got a plan; I'm disciplined; I'm going to be a success," and you stick to your guns, how is that making others feel about themselves?

Those on a health journey are not the only people who are trying to deal with change. Those on a plan just happen to be those who can implement the changes necessary to achieve better health. That leaves the remainder wanting a better body and improved health, but struggling with making the life changes necessary to achieve the result.

As scared as you are of making necessary changes in your life, others are just as scared. That often results in them becoming

Baiters because if they see others changing for the better, that would mean that they must change themselves. If that person is not ready to make those changes, it can make them feel resentful and bitter towards you for ruining their chocolate cake breakfast and poor health behaviors.

People don't want to see their friends turn down a drink or a piece of chocolate cake because that might mean that they must change. They will need to resolve the conflict within themselves to tackle change and may not be as ready as you were. Thus, these issues are about them, not you.

When dealing with Baiters, the best thing to remember is that it isn't about you as much as it is about them. You need to take their behaviors, actions, and comments for what they are: a camouflaged compliment that may appear as a dig or sabotage against you. Be proud; take note; and be sensitive; but stick to your guns.

Non-Believers

"The streets will flow with the blood of the non-believers."

Along your health journey, you will come across and will have to deal with plenty of non-believers.

Non-believers are like Haters and Baiters. The issues are very similar to the core social and psychological behaviors of human dynamics. Nobody was born a pure health aficionado. Health improvement is a process that must be honed based on habits and behaviors. A healthy lifestyle is the implementation of rock-solid, time-tested, and proven principles of success.

You have heard the stories of people losing a hundred pounds or more. People may want to believe that the reason they aren't healthy is because they didn't grow up with the right parents or best genetics. That is a common misconception, but that is not how the world works. It is natural to desire an easy path such as being born into a health-conscious family. But as many people demonstrate, it is not mandatory that you come from a great family situation or have perfect genetics.

Hard work along with the acquisition of skills over time is not something that many want to believe in, and that is what makes them "non-believers."

Those that implement a healthy lifestyle all must learn and implement the same skills as other health and wellness practitioners. They may do it in different ways or for different periods of time, but the core curriculum is similar for all healthy individuals.

Non-Believers are like those who hear you are on a diet and will lash out and say, "Oh, give it a week and you'll be back to eating chips and ice-cream."

Non-Believers don't want to see the permanent and beneficial change in others because it would rock their internal belief system. If they were forced to acknowledge that change was possible in somebody else, it would imply that change is possible within them (if they would only put in the effort to change). Since they are not willing to make changes within themselves, it only makes sense that they are Non-Believers with others who are attempting change.

Non-Believers tend to come across as Debbie-Downers or Negative-Neds. They won't have a single word of encouragement for you. Rather, they will express their internal belief system on you in hopes that you don't change. The non-believers will exhibit this behavior so that they don't feel bad about themselves for not making the effort to change.

You must remember that most of the people around you have similar backgrounds. They may have grown up in the same family, or the same neighborhood, attended the same schools, or work for the same company. There is typically a lot of common ground between you and your social circle. When you change, it rocks the order and stability of their known universe.

If everybody in your group is convinced that they could never become healthy and fit because of their employers, their genetics, their upbringing, or the government, and you come in and prove otherwise, that's a hard thing for them to come to grips with because it exposes the flaws in their belief system, thus creating internal conflict within them.

That will force many to either change themselves (highly doubtful) or create a loophole for their behavior system by stating that the success of someone else was due to luck or randomness. An attitude or belief such as this is a common behavioral response when somebody else isn't ready or willing to change. It feels safer and more comfortable for them to do nothing and wait for luck or randomness to change their reality. Unfortunately, life doesn't reward this type of inaction or stagnant behavior.

At the core of the social issues is a change in dynamics. Change is hard for everybody. Further, you need to acknowledge that your changes within yourself impact others whether it is directly or indirectly. If you are married or are a parent, and you are making healthy lifestyle changes, I can assure you that your new habits and behaviors will impact others, since you may want to eat healthier or do more activities. Spouses and children may not like that change and will fight you on it because they aren't ready for the change or don't see the benefits of change that you do.

A Strategy That Works For All Three

Whether you are dealing with Haters, Baiters, or Non-Believers, you may find it useful to respond to others by describing your new values and not the desired outcomes. When people nudge you to make poor health decisions, a lot of what they say falls into the, "Oh, come on, have a drink or eat a piece of cake and have some fun. You must live for today. You could be dead tomorrow," category. Some people can be rather pushy and aggressive in unexpected ways.

It may be helpful to state your new values positively, such as, "I want to improve myself," or express yourself regarding your feelings such as, "I am feeling excited about my progress." People have a much harder job when it comes to disputing or attacking feelings. What are they going to say, "No, you don't feel excited about making progress because I said so?" This approach accomplishes two objectives. It not only has a better chance of shutting down a pushy person, but it also reminds you of what you truly and deeply want to accomplish.

It is possible that you will lose friends as you improve your health to new and higher levels. Keep in mind that you can make new friends who share your desired values. You cannot get a do-over in life for many health problems. The days, weeks, and years will continue to expire and become the past. Friends, acquaintances, and co-workers will come and go, but you must ensure that your health and wellness efforts do not do the same. You must adhere to your personal set of values and principles.

To summarize and remind you once again before moving on, when you run into social dynamics with Haters, Baiters, and Non-Believers, you should take the instigation of others as a deeper hidden form of compliment. What it means is that people are taking notice of your progress at a level where it is impacting their behavior and emotions.

KEEP UP THE GOOD WORK!

Don't let others distract or discourage you from you own goals and objectives in life. Breakthrough health is possible when you stay true to yourself and your commitment to your own path.

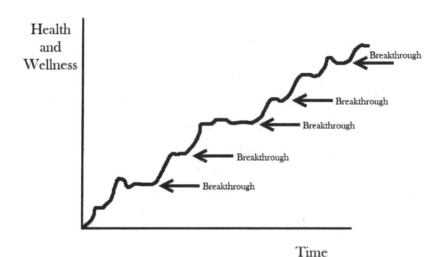

Bonus Chapter 2 – One Step At A Time

Most people struggle with their health. Unfortunately, the human brain isn't wired correctly for natural health success in modern society, so our brains are often working against us.

Humans are very social creatures, like all primates, in addition to being emotional. Humans are wired to seek out security, food, and reproduction. A lot of hardwiring is at play when humans make decisions that most people don't understand.

We Are Wired For Immediate Gratification

Corporations understand this when they market and advertise to us. They have become extremely effective and efficient in motivating us to make purchases of goods and services (like food and drinks) that we believe will make us happy, safe, or attractive.

Health improvement is a process and a progression of skills. It's important to think of it this way so that you don't get discouraged and quit before all the good factors start working for you. It's very similar to the overall education process that you went through as a child. In childhood education, you progress from one grade to the next by building off the skills previously acquired.

That's why I often say the following;

"Don't compare your Chapter 2 to somebody else's Chapter 14."

It's natural for you to want to be successful, and it's natural for you to want to look as successful as possible RIGHT NOW. Who isn't anxious to reap immediate benefits of being successful with their health and fitness right now? But there is a natural progression that must take place during the health improvement process.

In school, you wouldn't expect second graders to read, write, do math, and exhibit critical thinking like that of an eighth grader. Nor would you expect an eighth grader to perform on the same level as the average high school junior. In school, you progress systematically from one grade to another. There is a similar knowledge progression in health improvement.

However, society doesn't label those health progressions with grade levels for people to compare themselves against. In the real world of health and wellness, the grade levels are only known to the individual participants and reflected on their medical records as health metrics rather than grade levels. We must grade ourselves.

Unfortunately, you are not offered learning modules for health improvement during your formal public education. That does not mean that you cannot learn about health or wellness or that you cannot continually progress to higher levels during your lifetime. Fortunately, you can continue to learn and acquire more health improvement skills and knowledge over your entire lifetime. There are no age limits on health education.

You will have to come to terms with breaking the process down into smaller steps. Success comes when you focus on just one or two significant objectives at a time.

It's not reasonable (or possible) to learn everything there is on all facets of health and wellness, such as nutrition, or exercise, or recovery, all at once in a few short weeks. It is better to focus on one skill at a time, as opposed to doing a dozen items haphazardly or with poor execution.

A Lot To Learn – One Step At A Time

When you commit to a healthy lifestyle, you can't successfully implement too many changes at once. The best strategy is to choose one or two goals that you think will move the needle the most. Then focus. Track those items. Benchmark those items. Make notes of those items including what parts of them you can and can't control.

When you first start, there will be some aspects of the journey that you haven't yet mastered. You may not have accurate record keeping. You may not be good at choosing meal plans. You may not be good at using gym equipment. You may not be good at being disciplined about going to bed on a consistent schedule.

These are some of the steps, processes, and objectives that you will have to learn and apply as you implement a healthy lifestyle. There is nothing worrisome about your lack of natural ability in any area of health. What will make you special and different from everyone else is your ongoing commitment to learning and implementing the necessary skills in the areas that matter regarding health and wellness. But remember, you CAN do it. You can transform your life like many others before you. Sometimes the learning is slow and frustrating. But others have learned, and you can too.

Keep in mind though, when you commit to living a healthy lifestyle, something else will suffer. You can't be all things to all people, nor will you even be the same person anymore. But ultimately that's the point. If you wanted to be the same person, then you would be saying, "I'm fine being overweight, lethargic, and at high risk (or already dealing with) chronic diseases that were avoidable."

This process is about YOU, your results, and your personal transformation.

Don't fool yourself like most others who think that health is a one-time event like a fad diet that looks like this:

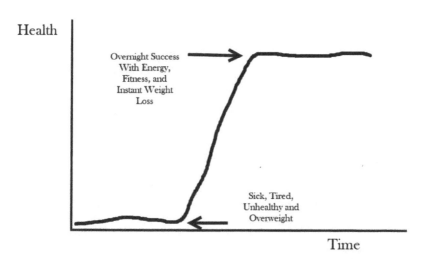

That isn't reality. Breakthrough health is a series of constant improvements that evolve as you learn more and apply more skills to your own life. Breakthrough health is a series of improvements as you master one phase of your life and move on to higher challenges and accomplishments.

Build
Momentum

Breakthroughs

Start Now

Track Results

Eat Healthy Foods

Sunshine and Fresh Air

Take A Deep Breath

Create Processes

CROWD OUT AND SUBSTITUTE

EXERCISE

DAILY

PROVEN PRINCIPLES

Just A Tiny Bit More Than Yesterday

Develop Better Habits

Avoid Sleep Destroyers

Simplify Your Life

Learn Your Hairpin Triggers

Morning Rocket Fuel

FOLLOW MENTORS

Visualize The Future You

Eat Out Wisely

Learn From YouTube

Reduce The Sugar

Have Fun While Exercising

NO BLUE LIGHTS BEFORE BED

Relax The Muscles

ADEQUATE SLEEP   Listen To A Good Podcast

Bonus Chapter 3 - Do Your Best

Life is hard. I want to share some insight with you. Life is hard for everybody. Life is hard at both ends of the social spectrum on wealth and health. Sure, people at the lower end of the social spectrum will say, "Yeah, but my life is harder because I don't have a lot of financial resources in my life." And that would be true. Their life is hard and will continue to be hard.

But even those who have progressed have a hard life because they are making a lot of sacrifices along the way. They are living with deferred gratification. They are living with deferred consumption. They are living with restraint. They are working very hard and giving up their free time in pursuit of individual financial and health goals. Constantly working to improve yourself and acting diligently is very hard to do, and that is exactly why most people don't do it. Doing nothing is the easiest route to take in life. The harder path is the one filled with work.

So, Why Aren't They Climbing?
Such a paradox leads to an interesting juncture in society because those at the lower end of the social scale will say, "But it's not as hard for those other people who have more." But if it is easier higher up the social ladder, why aren't they doing the things necessary to climb it? Why aren't others using their free time to read books, work overtime, get fit, handle potential failures, and even lose money while learning the skills? Why

aren't others trading their personal time for self-education? Why don't they strive for good grades in school? Why? They don't do those things and exhibit those behaviors because all those endeavors are HARD! That is the only reason people don't do them.

It will be hard no matter the route you take in life. If you want to be a success, your life will be hard. If you don't want to be a success, your life will of course, still be hard. Choose wisely and consciously.

No One Said It Would Be Easy

If you are committing to a life of success, then I encourage you to do your best. When you do your best, you won't live a life of regret.

Be aware that doing your best is a variable endeavor. None of us ever perform at maximum potential every second of every day. Sometimes you will get tired. Sometimes you will get frustrated. Sometimes you will get discouraged. Sometimes you will get distracted. Sometimes you will get sick. Sometimes somebody you love will need help.

In those circumstances, still do your best. Be honest and ask yourself, "Am I doing my best right now with my current situation?"

Trying your best and then being patient with yourself when you aren't performing to maximum capacity may sound contradicting. Many factors in life seem contradicting and paradoxical. However, life is not all about suffering. The purpose of life is not to strip all joy out of your existence. That is a wasted life.

A healthy lifestyle is a choice. The reason you make that choice is to be happier overall. You make that commitment and choice because you believe your life will be better overall as a healthy and fit individual than your life would be as a sick and unhealthy person. You make decisions, sacrifices, and trade-offs that improve the totality of your life, not diminish your overall existence.

The pursuit of health is a choice that is made to improve your life, not to destroy your life and sometimes there will be a fine line that you must not cross. There are countless people on this earth who work extremely hard seven days a week. They suffer as they work. They suffer with their personal relationships. They suffer as they progress through life. If you find yourself in a situation where most of your life involves suffering, then you are failing in life, and it's time to regroup and assess what is going wrong.

To do your best means putting in the time, the effort, and the energy into pursuits that are most meaningful to you. Happiness results when you make progress towards goals and objectives that are important to you. When you are moving towards goals that you want, your happiness will flourish. When you are moving away from goals that you value, your happiness is fleeting.

You have a right to be happy in life. You will find success in the pursuit of happiness when you do your best on the items that are most important to you.

Remember that a healthy lifestyle is something that should enhance your life and make you happier. You aren't doing this as personal punishment. Life isn't a contest on who can suffer and deny themselves the most. That isn't the goal. A healthy body allows you to do more in life, not less. It's just that few people realize this because they never had a health standard of excellence so that they could experience the benefits first hand.

Bonus Chapter 4 - Help Others

It is difficult to succeed without the help of others. Others before us have taken the time to write articles, write books, create tools, share wisdom, pass on mistakes, and carve a smoother path through thick forests of unproductivity.

We learn both from our first-hand experiences where you try techniques for yourself, and through the experiences of others who have come before you. There are plenty of successful individuals who have already figured out the process of health improvement and are willing to pass on their knowledge to those interested in learning.

You must remember that no matter where you are in your journey, there are others who are already many levels above you. Likewise, regardless of how little you are starting out with, there will be others who will still be many levels below you. You can obtain not only knowledge but encouragement, coaching, mentoring, and a helping hand from others who share common goals and pursuits. You in turn can also share, encourage, and help others with their pursuits.

You may think to yourself, "I can't help anybody because I don't know much or haven't yet accomplished much." But that is not true. The fact that you are seeking wisdom as you take steps towards improvement and start to implement new resources and ideas means that you are many steps ahead of others who are further back or stuck entirely.

You may worry what others will think if you make changes to your life. You may fear that they will resent you, or question you, or make fun of you. But on the other hand, you might have the power to inspire them. They may also desire a change. They may also be seeking knowledge and self-improvement. If that is the case, be sure to help others.

"When you learn, teach. When you get, give." – Maya Angelou

"While we teach, we learn." – Seneca

You are like those who surround you which means that most of the people with whom you associate with are probably around the same level of health as you are, and probably all striving to have more and show more success, just like you. You are likely very similar to others in your social circle.

Be sensitive to the fact that not everybody wants the same changes as you, nor are they on the same time frame as you. You have your individual path to follow. Forcing your newfound knowledge on others is not the desired intent of this exercise. Rather, it is to become aware that others around you might also be in search of positive personal changes regarding health and wellness, and it can be quite effective to work together in pursuit of common goals.

Many have the desire to get in better physical shape. Is it easier or harder when others around you are doing it together? Is it easier or harder when someone else is holding you accountable to your goals and achievements? Is it easier or harder when multiple people are in it together and sharing knowledge, experience, and feedback as to what is and isn't working?

If you wanted to improve your health, you would most likely find it is easier to meet a new friend who has similar goals as you do at a gym rather than at a local bar on a Wednesday night. Choose your hang out spots and social surroundings appropriately based on your desires and goals in life.

There is not a shortage of people who desire an improvement in their health and wellness. Most would love to be able to improve their health at a faster pace, or even just begin to build some momentum. Reach out and help others who can use a helping hand, words of encouragement, and empathy as they make mistakes, and help them celebrate their breakthroughs.

You will get more out of it than you can imagine.

"It's hard to soar like an eagle when you are hanging out with a bunch of turkeys all day."

Bonus Chapter 5 - Starting Over

Sometimes our biggest fear in life is starting over. This fear could relate to a big issue, or a smaller issue. However, starting over could also be a wonderful opportunity. If you tried something and it didn't work, then you must simply start over with another approach that may work more effectively.

"Insanity is doing the same thing over and over again and expecting different results." – Albert Einstein

It is time to progress to the next level. It may be long overdue in your life. It is time to give up on your ideals of perfection and a lucky winning lottery ticket to success. The path won't be a perfect one. It will be bumpy and rocky. It will have twists and turns.

Health improvement will not always be easy. Everything inside of you will be tempted to wait to get started or make the necessary changes tomorrow, next week, or next year. Your inner self will naturally want to procrastinate. Acting and moving forward with new processes is what you must do if you want to be successful and improve your health.

If you feel nervous and unsure, that is natural. You are experiencing normal emotions. You must take a leap of faith and commitment. Have faith that you will create a better life for yourself and move past your current levels. But you must also have the commitment to make that faith a reality. Trust in yourself that you can make changes one step at a time, which will lead to forward progress towards your health goals and objectives.

When you learn and implement the required changes in your life, you will begin to get the results and transformation that you seek. You will slowly become a different person.

But you must not wait. Act, do your best, accumulate knowledge, and progress to the next level. Find the courage to push yourself out of your current state and level. Once you stop dreaming and start doing, your life will have a fascinating way of falling into place as you get results and experience a transformation.

YOU CAN DO IT

OTHERS HAVE PROVEN IT COULD BE DONE

MAKE YOUR MARK ON THE WORLD

LIVE IN PURSUIT OF YOUR GOALS

About The Author

Paul Kindzia is a writer, health and wellness advocate, portfolio manager, wealth advisor, and CEO of Kindzia Investments, Inc. a registered investment advisory practice outside of Atlanta, GA. His personal mission is to teach others how to improve their health and wealth and improve their happiness.

Paul is a certified public accountant with an undergraduate degree from the State University of New York at Buffalo (1992). He also holds an MBA in corporate finance from the State University of New York at Buffalo (1994). He is a member of the American Institute of Certified Public Accountants.

Paul is a Certified Financial Planner (CFP®).

He is an avid reader and writer with an ever-expanding personal library. He has a love of nature, science, animals, and the ocean.

Paul is a proponent of maintaining personal health and wellness. He enjoys an active and healthy lifestyle and is a 13-time Ironman triathlon finisher. He has also completed numerous marathons including but not limited to the San Diego Rock N' Roll Marathon, Nashville Country Music

Marathon, Disney Marathon, New York City Marathon, and his personal favorite the Marine Corp Marathon in Washington, D.C.

Paul lives outside of Atlanta, GA with his family and an ever-expanding pack of rescue dogs. He is an animal lover at heart and the family often volunteers with English Springer Rescue America (ESRA) or helping some stray cats.

He also enjoys behavioral finance, investments, endurance athletics, martial arts, music, video production, making sushi and has a tremendous passion for jiu-jitsu, fishing, and scuba diving.

You can keep up with him at **www.paulkindzia.com**

For additional valuable information including free resources, please visit our website at:

www.paulkindzia.com

Be sure to check out our other publications

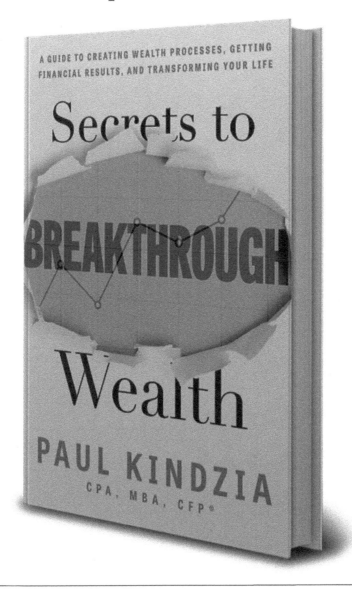